Letter to Louis

Letter to Louis

ALISON WHITE

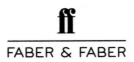

FABER & FABER

First published in 2018
by Faber & Faber Limited
Bloomsbury House
74–77 Great Russell Street
London WC1B 3DA

Typeset by Faber & Faber Limited
Printed and bound by CPI Group (UK) Ltd, Croydon, CR0 4YY

The right of Alison White to be identified as author of this work
has been asserted in accordance with Section 77 of the Copyright,
Designs and Patents Act 1988

A CIP record for this book
is available from the British Library

ISBN 978–0–571–33563–3

2 4 6 8 10 9 7 5 3 1

For Louis, Greg, Tasha, Jack

'Where are you going today?' says Pooh:
'Well, that's very odd 'cos I was too.'
'Let's go together,' says Pooh, says he.
'Let's go together,' says Pooh.

'Us Two' by A. A. Milne

ZERO

The doctor is pacing around my trolley, checking the trace. He's threatening to deliver you here and now in this waiting room. *Is it really so serious? You'd think I'd feel more.* I try to keep calm. I take long deep breaths like my father taught me years ago when I couldn't sleep at night. I watch the clock above the door. The silver hands move slowly around its face and I hope that Greg will appear. He'll get home, get the messages, get here in time.

⌣

You are lifted out wriggling: no sound, no cry, away from my sight, lost behind doctors in the far corner of the room as I lie paralysed. The anaesthetist whispers into my ear from behind.

'It's a boy,' he says.

All I can see is the dulled green cotton of the operation sheet placed across my chest. It has drooped lower, one more inch and I will see the slice, my body open.

The blue-dressed doctors are busy; four of them crowd around you under the strip-lights but no one is speaking. And then you are gone. You disappear to the sound of a foghorn, a booming box on wheels.

'Where is he going?'

'Intensive care,' a voice filters in.

The two obstetricians remain. They stand over me, studying what is hidden from my view. One is looking down concentrating, moving her hands in a sewing motion.

⌣

It is hot, so very hot. Am I in a cupboard? A fan is churning the air but it isn't helping me, my mouth is dry and parched, and I feel feverish. What is this room? There is medical equipment, a broom, but no windows. I am alone in this strange room and a nurse keeps appearing and disappearing as I vomit and bleed. A pain has begun to throb in my numbed waist. There is a syringe of yellow liquid attached to my hand: I feel its cold texture trickle in. The door shakes, the handle lowers and Greg bursts into the room. He's clutching something; it's a blurred blob on a Polaroid. I beam at him.

'Greg! We have a baby boy – a "Louis" – and you thought it would be a girl!'

He doesn't smile back. He collapses onto the end of the bed and his shoulders heave.

'It's okay', I say, 'everything's okay.'

⌣

I don't recognise the sound. My mouth is open but the noise I can hear is distorted; high pitched but deep, it sounds like a cow. It feels like my blood has turned to mercury and is pouring rapidly through my veins and spreading out across the floor. I'm trying to scream Greg's name for help.

The shower tray is cold and hard. The nurse helps me up and into a wheelchair, back to the hospital bed where I have been lying for the last sixteen hours since you were born.

I've been feverish all night, drifting in and out of sleep, vomiting, feeling throbbing pain in the wound. Behind my closed eyelids I'd seen your head, your body being lifted out wriggling, your eyes glued closed, your tiny mouth gasping but making no sound. Later I will know that your heart was not beating. You were dying as you were born.

I'm in a chair. The nurse wheels me out of the lift and presses the buzzer.

'It's mum for one of the new ones,' she says.

The lock releases and I'm wheeled through, turned down a corridor. I can feel the warm air on the bare skin of my back, between the ties of the gown. I'm clutching a sick bowl. It's been twenty hours since you were born.

I'm going to see you.

I'm wheeled past the notice board with babies displayed. I don't register it today. That will come later when I will hover here waiting for the doctors' round to be over. I will stare at pictures of babies going home with their mothers, and tremble as I block out the board alongside showing those who don't.

5

Will I be able to tell which you are?

I'm wheeled through another set of double doors and the heat hits me. Blinds are pulled down across all of the windows, fluorescent lights shine from the ceiling and clear plastic incubators line the room in two rows.

I can see at the end a perfect baby; its porcelain skin seems to glow. It's large: it must be full term, and is rolled onto its side, unmoving, eyes closed. A man and a woman stand stationary next to it; their eyes are cast down and I sense there is no hope. I learn in that instant that we don't stare. We don't talk to each other in here.

There are three in a row to my left all the same size, teeny ones all on their stomachs, positioned like rabbits with upturned bottoms cushioned in nappies, knitted hats that could fit on an egg. *Are you the one with the tuft of black hair?* No, she has wheeled me past.

Now she has stopped.

I would not have chosen you.

You are tiny. You look like a flattened frog. Your thin arms and legs are splayed outwards and wrapped in tape, weighted down by splints holding wires that thread into your veins. Your blond hair seems woven and is stuck to your head, your golden skin covered in down. Your eyes are tightly closed. I can't see the rest of you. There are two large corrugated tubes, one green and one white. There's a pipe in your mouth. There is white padding and sticking tape. I can't see your nose, your mouth, most of your cheeks. The pipe is pumping and pumping. Your whole body is shaking from head to toe. Your

6

chest is expanding, stretching your skin tightly across your rib cage then dropping.

Circular pads are stuck to your chest and I hear bleeping, your heart beating. To the right I see a machine, a squiggle, your heart rate. It suddenly stops and an alarm pierces my ear. You try to lift your splinted arm and I know, even now on first meeting, that you are trying to swat the sound away. A nurse steps forward, presses a pad down on your chest, checks the machine, stops the alarm that's triggering constantly, making you jump.

'Hello, my name is Natalie. I will be watching over your son.'

I like her immediately; she is warm and motherly, with dark patches under her eyes and the smell of coffee on her breath. *Someone is here for you.* I try to smile but instead I'm convulsing, vomit is rising out of my stomach onto my gown. I heave again and fluid erupts with a force that sends it splattering over the floor.

The alarm is triggering. You are jumping again and I'm leaving you. They are wheeling me hurriedly away.

~

A middle-aged doctor rushes past; he stops.

'Are you Louis's parents? I'm Dr Nook.'

We nod.

I'm still feeling queasy, my eyesight is blurring. *Oh no, am I going to pass out?*

The doctor tilts his head, running his hand through his thick black hair. He looks like he's not had much sleep.

'Your son has been giving us a run for our money.'

The doctor seems wired. His voice is nasal, his words staccato like gunfire; I can barely follow.

'You're lucky; we've got the oscillating ventilator free. Your son needs to be shaken to stop his lungs from sticking together. The steroids should have helped his lungs to mature but there was no time to wait for them to work before we had to deliver. So now we have to shake him and pump him with air in order to breathe.'

'Will he be okay?'

That's Greg. His voice sounds fuzzy.

'Your son's condition has to be taken minute by minute, hour by hour right now.'

My head is starting to spin. The doctor turns away but then he turns back again, taking a breath.

'One other thing: we are sending some of Louis's blood away for genetic testing just to be sure he is normal. I've detected three congenital anomalies: a hypospadias, a single umbilical vein and thirteen ribs. These are all very common and I'm not concerned at all but as there are three it's our practice to check.'

He's gone. His footsteps clip quick down the corridor, stop and turn through the intensive care doors. An alarm rings out, is cut dead. The doors swing shut.

In my bed I'm wheeled into a lift, down and out again, along the corridor and through swing doors into East Wing. A ward sister walks towards me as I enter.

'I'm ever so sorry. I'm aware of your circumstances but I'm afraid we can't give you your own room right now: there's been a spate of deliveries; you'll have to stay in the main ward for now. I'll move you as soon as I get the opportunity.'

Beaming visitors are huddled around beds, and past their shoulders I glimpse mothers propped up with pillows holding their swaddled babies, displaying them to their audience. I'm wheeled to an open cubicle with an empty bed and am asked to swap over. Shifting my body weight, I can feel a tug, the stitches pulling the skin, my wound starting to ooze as I hear my name.

'Alison! What on earth are you doing here?'

I turn my head to see Nicola. She's standing fully clothed with a baby in her arms. Nicola is an acquaintance, she was two months ahead of me and we'd been sharing progress whenever we'd met on the street.

'This is Matthew, isn't he perfect?'

I'm trying to nod.

'What are you doing here – you're not due yet?'

'I've had a baby boy – his name's Louis; he's up in intensive care.'

We both look at Matthew; there's nothing more to be said. Then Nicola speaks in her awkwardness.

'Oh my god, how dreadful, I couldn't cope with that.'

There's another nurse. She is tickling my breasts. The blood has drained from my face and I can feel bile rising from my stomach into my throat. She doesn't seem to notice my revulsion. My breasts are rock hard, skin stretched over solid what? What is in there? *God they hurt.*

'You need to extract some milk for your wee bairn. This first milk is the royal jelly.'

Oh shit this is hideous. She is gently pattering her pudgy white fingers on the skin, lightly tickling. She must be trying to mimic a baby's hand. She's stopped and stood back, thank goodness.

'Now here's the machine for you to borrow. You need to turn it on like this and attach the suction pump to your breast and screw the bottle onto it here.'

I'm confused.

'There aren't many of these at the hospital but you qualify and it should be easier for you than hand pumping. Now you must get started straight away. You'll need to ask your husband to get you a steriliser for all the parts.'

'Oh.' *Steriliser? Where from?*

'Here's some bottles. Write your hospital number onto these labels, put them on your bottle and bring them up to the ward freezer. We don't want them accidentally giving your royal jelly to the wrong wee bairn now, do we?'

She talks in a voice that is girlishly hushed. Her hair is mouse-brown and she's tall with pink moist lips. She seems different to the other nurses – lonely. Although I feel sorry for her, my overriding feeling is disgust. I don't want her to touch my breast.

'I'm going to go and get you a sheet that your son has been lying on; its scent will help to stimulate your milk.'

She returns with a brushed-cotton sheet. There are blood-stains.

'This is your son's, give it a good smell.'

She stands there.

Please just go away, will you?

I've never been admitted to a hospital before: this is to-tally alien to me, the bright lights, the heat, the staff, these procedures. This isn't what I learnt in the antenatal class. There's another woman in this small room tucked down the corridor from the intensive care unit; we are both in hospital gowns, pale and silent. We haven't acknowledged each other yet. I don't think we will.

'Now you need to go on the pump at least every four hours both day and night, preferably try three hours to start with, that will help to get your milk flowing, it will help to give your baby the best possible chance.'

This is all that I can do for you right now.

⌢

'Doctor, last night as I sat watching Louis I touched his hand through the incubator' – *rested his tiny finger the size of a matchstick on mine* – 'and he opened his eyes for the first

11

time and I thought I could see terror there. Could this be so?'

The doctor jerks backwards suddenly in his chair, tilts his head and looks at me with his ageing angular face.

'I'm a doctor, we don't do feelings,' he says abruptly. 'He's on morphine, so he should not be in any pain. I think only about keeping him alive.'

He pauses, sighs, speaks again softly.

'You need to be aware that this is going to be like taking a rollercoaster ride. Hopefully in a few months' time you will take your baby home with you.'

⁓

'Do you have his birth certificate yet?' a nurse asks gently. There's something in her tone – why the urgency? I'm sitting by the incubator staring at you, looking at every detail of your body. I feel happy; you are five days old and I'm thinking how well you are looking.

'Could you come into my office a moment, please?'

My heart lifts. I like these occasional discussions with Dr Thompson on your progress. I'm still feeling elated since our last chat when he told me your ultrasound brain scan was exceptionally promising, no bleeds at all.

'Your baby is giving us serious concern. We believe he may be developing necrotising enterocolitis. He has not passed any stools yet and his stomach is grossly distended, these are the usual signs. There is a real chance his gut will rupture in the next couple of hours, with little chance of survival if it does. You need to be prepared for what might happen very soon.'

I am plummeting down a black hole. My arms are outstretched, fingers splayed, slicing channels down the clay-slimed walls. I'm hurtling faster and faster, down and down. There is no end.

I go down to the ward and find the telephone for patients. Holding the receiver tight to my ear I drop coins into the box. I'm calling my uncle Len, a paediatrician. I've been calling him every day since you were born.

I'm having difficulty speaking through my sobs.

'They are seriously worried about Louis. They think that his gut might rupture and he might die. I haven't even held him.'

I'm sobbing uncontrollably.

He talks to me gently, asks simple questions. He takes a practical stance.

'Look, you are on day five and it's a medical fact your hormones will be plummeting. You would be feeling mixed emotions even without these terrible circumstances. You must take some deep breaths. Go back up to his incubator and sit by his side. That will make you feel more in control.'

I sit motionless by your incubator.

13

Now all I can see is your stomach swollen. Your belly button is black and flattened and your skin is stretched taut over your abdomen; like a crust on a baking pie, it looks like it will split open at any moment.

The room is peaceful; it is 'quiet time', just the bleeps of the monitors, the babies all sleeping. The porcelain baby has gone. Its incubator disappeared from the room some time in the night. I think of those parents and I feel pain and a sense of dread. The little chapel set back off the stairwell. *Please, no, don't let it be you too.*

There are sounds of hospital activity from the corridor outside. A nurse appears beside us, begins to clean your mouth with cotton buds, removing scum that has formed around the ventilator pipe.

'Would you like to help?'

She's kind. I dip the bud into a tiny bottle of sterilised water; gently wipe your dry, white-crusted dribble away.

'This isn't usually allowed but I need to change the sheet, would you like to lift him? Be very careful with the wires.'

My heart leaps. I place my hands through the windows into your womb and slide them carefully under you and gently lift. Our skins are touching at last. The beat of my heart is pulsing in my hands, and I do not want this moment to end. I can feel your fragile weight, our warm skins melting together.

'Place him down now.'

Her voice filters in and as I slowly lower you, thick black treacle-like globules ooze from your bottom, drop onto the sheet.

I'm here at last, you can let go now. Doctor, doctor, he's going to be okay.

The nurse tuts. 'I'm going to have to change it all over again.'

I'm soaring high above the hospital rooftop, racing through the grey clouds, further and further, the dense clouds are thinning, seeping light, I burst through them into blue sky.

⌣

'Len, Louis is going to be okay, he's just done a poo. The doctor is saying the main danger is over, the x-ray has come back clear.'

Years later your great-uncle Len enjoyed telling me how he'd walked around his hospital that afternoon with a grin stretched across his face. A colleague eventually asked him, 'So why are you looking so pleased?' And he'd answered, 'Because a little boy in Scotland has just done a poo.'

⌣

Natalie has gone. She is standing by another incubator in the intensive care room. I almost run.

'Natalie, why aren't you by Louis?'

'Alison, please.' Her shadowed face is smiling; she takes

my hand. 'Do not be sad, this is good news. Your son is no longer the most critical here, be glad.'

~

There have been emotional phone calls in the evenings between Greg and my mother while I have been sleeping at the hospital. Now your grandparents, Spike and Mary, have come up from Sheffield to see you. I lead them down the corridor towards the intensive care room. As we get closer I notice Spike has fallen back. As we reach the double doors to the intensive care room I stop and demonstrate how we must carefully cleanse our hands and arms with antiseptic lotion. Spike's hands stay down by his side and he tilts his body to lean against the glass-sectioned wall that looks into your room of incubators.

'I'll just stay here,' he says quietly looking down.

'But you won't get to see him.' There's surprise in my voice.

'We don't want to overcrowd him right now.'

'But Dad?'

Spike's face is pale. This is not like him. We leave him standing in the corridor and I take Mary into the room, over to your plastic bubble. We stare into your incubator and Mary's eyes fill with tears. As we turn to leave Mary whispers, 'Your father, he can't cope with this.'

Later as Spike pats my shoulder to say goodbye he says quickly, 'I'm sorry, Ali. I don't want to get close to him, in case he doesn't make it.'

16

Spike's sister died at the age of fourteen; she dropped down dead in the street from a brain haemorrhage. It was Spike who had to tell his parents. I know those memories have engulfed him.

Later you two will become peas in a pod. Later Spike will come up frequently to visit to help us to care for you. Later he will do anything, just anything, for you.

Seven days have passed. I've stepped out of the hospital. Cold autumn air enters my lungs, I feel its cool presence swirl into my brain and it is as if I am waking from a dream. I stand in the hospital car park, my coat wrapped over my black pyjama bottoms. We need to get to the birth register office to register your name.

The car is heading down a familiar street near the hospital. The tenements on each side are leaning in towards me, their red sandstone wrapping around the car. I grip the handle of the door tight. I feel like I'm in a time capsule passing a world I no longer know. I can feel the throbbing of my wound and I try not to panic. I close my eyes and I see you in your bubble under those harsh fluorescent lights, jumping, startled by the beeping, the triggering of the alarms.

In the waiting room we sit on a hard varnished bench until we are called into an office. A stout, dark-haired woman is sitting behind a desk. She takes both of our names.

'And your son, whose name is he to have?'

'We were thinking of giving him a double barrelled name, both of ours.'

She looks perturbed.

'Oh no, no, no, you don't want to go doing that, that'll mean that you,' she points at me, 'are in one place,' she swings her arm to point at Greg, 'and you are in another and your son, your poor wee boy, will be somewhere entirely different.'

We look at each other; Greg rolls his eyes.

'Well, let's have yours then,' I whisper. 'We'll have your surname.'

She overhears me.

'Oh no, no, no, you don't want to go doing that if you're not married; I'd definitely recommend the mother's name under these circumstances.'

She says it as if these circumstances are rare, with a relish. I'm really not up to this right now. I just need to get back to the hospital. I can feel my breasts swelling with milk; I need to get onto that pump.

Greg leans towards me. 'Just do your name. I don't mind, it really doesn't matter.'

'Okay, put it in my name.' I sigh as the words leave my mouth. *Doesn't she realise you are our son, both of ours?*

We pause outside on the steps; I'm holding your birth certificate in my hand.

'She was a nutball, what was that all about?'

'She didn't seem to understand we're together.'

I face Greg.

18

'Let's get married.'
Which of us said that?

The tube is stuck with masking tape across your cheek. It pokes through your nostril and disappears. I know it is resting down in your stomach; it must feel strange. The nurse measured you carefully, your length from your stomach to your nose, cut a length of tube and pushed it down your nostril, down your throat as you gagged. Now she is back with a bottle of my milk in her hand, in the other a plastic syringe. She draws out some milk from the bottle with the syringe then attaches it to the end of the tube. She squirts it down into your stomach. Now she washes the milk that's been left in the tube down there too, this time using sterilised water to push it through. It's all in your stomach. She studies her watch. She doesn't wait long before she sucks it all up again. She's using the same syringe, attaches it back on the tube and pulls slowly back with the plunger as it sucks up the contents. I see milk appear, sliding up the tube; it's tinged pink. *Is that blood? At least it's not green and pussy like last time.* She squirts some onto a piece of litmus paper.

'There now,' she says, looking pleased, 'he's starting to digest his food; now his feeds can be gradually increased. This is a very good sign.'

They've sent me home. It is ten days since you were born and they need my bed. I arrive back to a cold, quiet flat. I find a table and take it into our bedroom and place the milking machine on top. I put an armchair by its side; I'll be sitting in this day and night. I can't speak right now. I've lost the ability to speak to anyone but Greg and Len and the doctors and nurses up at the hospital. Greg fields the phone calls, he tells family and friends how you are doing each day. I can't. I've become mute. A fear like a suffocating fog seems to expand in my lungs with each day of being away from you; I need to get back to the ward, be by your side.

Greg has compiled a soothing music tape for me to listen to. Greg has a gift with music, his own and sourcing others. While I've been sleeping at the hospital he has come home and made up a collection of songs that he thinks will help me. It does, it helps to calm me, unfreeze my fear, release me briefly from the terror of us falling, you leaving this world. My mind cannot concentrate on anything other than you. I cannot read, I cannot watch a film, I cannot write, but as the music seeps into my mind I find I can relax a little. I start to read poetry. I find this helps me too. Suddenly I don't feel alone; I feel understood, as poets share their own pain.

We develop a routine that results in us being up at the hospital most of the day and evening with brief trips home to the pump. We start with a morning visit timed for after the doctors' round, one in the afternoon, one in the evening, and one late at night just before going to sleep. Greg sings to you in your incubator then, he sings in a quiet deep voice, he sings, 'I was born under a wand'rin star', and I'm sure that your body relaxes, that you enjoy the deep vibrations.

The autumnal light is golden; the leaves are turning yellow, orange and red as I watch the squirrels gathering their nuts for the winter. I am filled with hope. One day, one day next autumn, you and I will be watching the squirrels hand in hand.

~

It's early morning and I'm carrying bottles of my breast milk over to the ward freezer: my day's collection. I spot the male nurse with the goggly eyes. I've asked him for bottles before and he only gives me three at a time. *That's not going to get me very far.* I keep having to ask for more. I wish I could help myself from the store and not keep having to ask. I try to time my visits for when one of the competent nurses is around but damn it's him.

'Ah, it's Ermintrude.'

Moron. Breathe.

And now I've missed seeing you, I'm not allowed in. It's nine in the morning and the doctors' round has started. Any parents in the intensive care room are asked to leave; we hover by the notice board waiting for news, watching the doctors through the glass pane in the wall, watching them move from one incubator to the next, picking up the clip board hanging on the end of each frame, studying the notes. They will be deciding the best course of action for you today. You are off the oscillating ventilator now and onto the CPAP ventilator. I can tell you don't like it; you try to pull it out sometimes.

I watch through the pane as a nurse is asked to lift you then places you back down. The feeding tube has coiled under your cheek. I can see you're wriggling but no one has noticed. I know it is hurting. You are trying to lift the weight of your head, move it off the tube but you can't and I can't go to you.

At last the round is over and I'm back by your side. I've scrubbed my hands, my arms; my reddened skin is becoming rough from the frequency but I mustn't risk an infection. I gently take the weight of your head to lift and turn your face the other way. Your cheek is indented. You stop wriggling but your eyes remain closed, scrunched up tight. *Is it the brightness of the fluorescent light overhead?* I go to the store cupboard and find a white cotton sheet and place it over your incubator; it diffuses the light, lessens the glare. I see your face relax, your eyes unscrew, opening to show glistening black pools. You stare out to the side and I bend down, gazing in at you. Your eyes are glazed but your face looks calm. I feel calm flood through me too. *There, that's better for you.* The light returns in a flash, your eyes scrunch shut.

'It's not night-time.'

The junior doctor strides away, the sheet in her hand.

We are starting to get to know the personalities of the doctors and nurses in here; I suppose this comes with time, you've been here for nearly a month now.

Dr Thompson leads the team. He is calm, intelligent and thoughtful and he has my absolute respect; he appears to have everyone's in here. The nurses mention him as they go about their work.

'Och he saves so many of the sick babes in here.'

'He's just an amazing man.'

'Here comes God,' they whisper, keeping their heads lowered, becoming bashful if he stops and speaks.

Often after the doctors' round he pops back to speak with me while I'm sitting by your incubator.

'And how does mother think Louis is today?'

And I tell him.

He values my opinion, not that I can tell the things that a doctor can see.

'I always think it is best to ask the mother, she has been watching over her baby – she often notices the first signs.'

He's hovering.

'We are concerned about Louis. His breathing is laboured; see how his chest is pulling up under his ribs? He has what is called a patent ductus, an open valve in his heart. All babies have this but they usually close during the birthing process. Because Louis was premature and delivered by caesarean section this hasn't happened. Fluid is entering his lungs and I can see that he is struggling. It may be that he requires an operation but I'm reluctant to do this right now as he would only have a fifty-fifty chance of survival.'

He stares me directly in the eye. I flinch. I look down into your incubator and see your chest sucking up under your ribs.

'I need you to watch over him carefully. Come and tell me if you see any change.'

A man in green scrubs appears behind the doctor.

'Ah Bill. I'm glad you could get over here. This is the wee boy I'm concerned about.'

The surgeon puts a stethoscope to your chest.

'Yes, I think we should operate; I can fit him in. Do him first thing in the morning if you'd like?'

'I'd like a little more time, thank you. Can I speak with you again shortly?'

'No problem at all, let me know when you've decided and I'll find a slot.'

Dr Thompson explains. 'You see, surgeons always like to operate. That is because they are surgeons. Some may call me conservative but I like to wait a little. Louis is under three pounds, he has low reserves and there is still the possibility the ductus may close. I would like to go for the conservative option: we are going to starve him of food, give the bare minimum of fluid to help protect his lungs from filling, and then we'll wait for a few weeks in the hope it might spontaneously close itself. I think the odds of Louis's survival would be better.'

He has gone. How many things can happen to you? A

crater has opened just when I thought you were through it all.

~

You are four weeks old and we are explaining our situation to the vicar. *Is he a vicar?* We are inside the church across the road from our flat. He asks us a few questions and it's quickly clear we don't fit the church's criteria: neither of us is religious.

'Well, this will be my last marriage as I am leaving the church for another vocation. I think you will be the perfect couple to end with.'

We have to wait two weeks before the ceremony can be performed.

~

Between the hospital and our flat is a section of street that contains an odd collection of small shops. Above the shops are flats that look down onto the busy main road; their windows are streaked with black dust and their net curtains are shabby.

I've been walking along this street many times since I came out of hospital. Near the end of the street is a shop with a metal grille over its window, and in the centre of the window is a mannequin displaying a gold Chinese dress that I always stare at. Every time that I pass this shop I hope that it will be open but it is always in darkness. I've tried the door a number of times even though there was no point.

Today on this autumn afternoon when I leave the hospital the sky is heavy and grey, its light has been squeezed away like a rag wrung free of water. But as I walk down the street with the shops I can feel my heart lift; in the distance, through the grille of the coveted shop, I can see a small bright ball of light. As I get closer the ball becomes a shining bare light bulb hanging down from the central ceiling rose. I try the shop door again but it is still locked, so I raise up my hand and knock hard on the door with my fist. A stooped Chinese man wearing steel-rimmed glasses opens the door.

'Madam. I'm sorry, we are wholesale.'

'It's the dress . . . '

'Yes?'

'. . . in your window. I'm getting married next week and I wondered if I could try it on?'

The man hesitates.

'Ah, well, we don't have a changing room. There is a toilet.'

'Oh, that's fine. Can I see if it fits me?'

He allows me to squeeze into his shop filled with cardboard boxes and I help him to take the dress off the mannequin.

'I'm afraid I do not have a mirror,' he says.

I slip the dress on in the toilet and step out into the shop.

'What do you think?'

His kind face breaks into a smile.

'It fits you.'

Greg is going to wear his grandfather's suit, so we are sorted except for the rings.

No one is coming to the wedding; we are having the ceremony between visits to see you. I'm still finding it difficult to speak to anyone outside of the hospital so it seems a sensible plan. Mary is tearful.

'Are you sure you don't want anyone to come? I could get on a train?'

'No, honestly, Mum, I need to be up at the hospital; we can celebrate another time.'

Jamie, Greg's musician friend, has also been asking to come to the wedding, offering to take some photographs for us.

'No,' Greg explains. 'I'm sorry, Jamie, but no one's coming – if I let one then how can we not let more?'

⁓

I am sitting beside your incubator while you sleep. Dr Thompson comes into the room.

'I hear you're getting married on Friday, Alison?'

'Yes, I am.' I smile.

'I just wanted to let you know that I've been wondering about that heart operation for wee Louis. I don't really think we can wait any longer for the valve to close. I've been discussing it with colleagues and we were thinking of going ahead with the operation on Friday, but the nurses have just told me your news.' His face has creased into a smile. 'So I think I'll postpone it just a little bit longer.'

I leap up. 'Oh no, please don't delay for this. Do what's right for Louis. We don't have to get married; it's not as important as this.'

'Well, I'm going to think about it some more.'

A little while later he returns.

'You know, I think I am going to wait just a little bit longer. Louis seems to be doing very well today.'

Louis, Louis, you are?

⁓

It's Friday morning and we drive up to the hospital. The nurses crowd around us.

'Let's take a wee picture of you and Louis. Don't you look smashing?'

I hold you in my arms. Your eyes are closed and your oxygen tube is running into your nose. You look very well today.

'Here you are, hen, a card for you.'

I open the card. Inside it says, 'To my Mummy and Daddy on your wedding day', and there are your feet printed in gold.

As we drive home, I speak aloud.

'You know, maybe we should have a photo?'

Greg's on the telephone immediately, but Jamie doesn't answer.

'If you get this message we're getting married at noon at the church opposite our flat. A photo would be good after all.'

We stand outside the church; it's cold but the sky is clear. The vicar is wearing a bishop's hat. I'm a little confused. *What religion are we getting married into?* I don't dare to ask.

'As you are on your own with no relatives, you may as well walk down the aisle together. Walk slowly down until you reach the altar and then I will take your vows. After that, maybe you can say a poem or a few words to each other if you wish.'

The church is actually a cathedral and stately in size. *Why does Glasgow have more than one cathedral? Is that something to do with his hat?* We walk slowly down the aisle past empty wooden pews and magnificent arching columns that reach up towards stained-glass windows set into the carved stone walls. The curving roof above my head seems to be rising higher and higher and in the distance I can see an elaborately embroidered cloth draping the altar and the vicar standing beside it in his white cassock and sash. His gaze rises up to the ceiling and then lowers to face us, his benign smile encouraging us forwards. We are halfway down the aisle and I can feel the presence of my family all around, as if they are there in the pews. I can sense them nodding and smiling, willing me on. I am shaking, my heart is lifting and my lips are trembling. The enormous wooden door behind us creaks, and then silence booms. I don't look back. But then I hear a sound, a high-pitched whistle, a tune. *That's Jamie!* Music echoes through the building, swirls around us as we walk.

'Here comes the bride.'

Tonight I pour my milk for you down the sink. We celebrated our wedding with a meal and some alcohol – I can't let that be given to you. I stare out of the bathroom window and watch snowflakes falling. They had started falling earlier as we crossed George Square and flagged a taxi, came up to see you at midnight before going to bed. I took it as a good sign, this beautiful flurry of flakes on our wedding night. Now it is three in the morning. Outside is a muffled stillness, there's no sound of traffic over our rooftop from the Great Western Road. I look up and the sky is dense white, the flakes are falling with such frequency that they are barely separated as they pass the bathroom window. I look down and watch them covering our communal back garden. All has become white: the walls, lawn, hedges, bins, the flowerbeds are hiding under their bed sheets in the depths of this night.

A few nights later I wake in a panic and come to see you in the middle of the night. It's quiet up here at this time. They dim the lights at night-time and bubble wrap lies over you to keep you warm, but the bleeps still sound. There's a different type of nurse on duty: older, sadder, quieter. There is one who is cruel. She makes nasty little comments directed at the sleeping babies. We try to make sure we are with you when her shift is on.

There are all kinds of personalities among the nurses: kind ones, friendly ones, chatty ones, forgetful ones, bored or unhappy ones, intelligent and gentle ones, some doing far more work than others.

Some of the nurses open up to me as I sit by your incubator.

'Oh, I could never have a baby myself. What would you want one of those for?' a nurse called Karen says, laughing; she says it with a funny shrug but she clearly means it. She always chatters as she works, letting me into her world.

'You see, hen, all you parents are different. Some of you mothers, like you for instance, sit by your weans day in day out, but others, well, they won't even come into the room. There was this one woman . . .'

Karen pauses; she's just changed your sheet and she's put the dirty one down on a table and has turned towards me.

'She had her wee one in intensive care but she never came in. She would stand outside over there, watching us through the glass of the wall but never saying a word, and she always turned away when I came out of the room. I thought she was a right stuck-up cow. But then one day as I came out of the door she spoke to me. Her voice was shaking and she asked me, "How's my baby?" And I told her, "He's doing well." Well, she had started to shake. She told me she was too scared to come into the room. So I sat her down and told her not to worry, that it would be good for her and good for the baby. She told me she was scared to love him in case he died and I told her it was far better if she let him know she was there and that she loved him whatever happened. So she came with me into the room and I helped her to hold her baby. She came every day after that, until it died that is, poor thing. I learnt something then: you can never tell what you parents are thinking and feeling inside. And just to think I'd thought she was a stuck-up cow at first.'

Karen picks up your sheet and is moving away.

Take deep breaths, deep breaths.

⌒

It is Monday morning, you are seven weeks old and I am rushing down the corridor; I can hear the cries of the babies as I pass each of the rooms. They call it 'the torture hour' and they say this gleefully. I want to get to you in time, to be there to gently wake you, but I'm too late. I reach the end of the ward and turn into your own personal room. You've got an infection; you're in isolation right now. I can hear you screaming and I see *her*, the cruel nurse, holding the heel of your foot. She has come and stabbed the needle into your heel, not even bothering to wake you first. She's squeezing the blood and it's dropping into a test tube that's nearly half full. She drops your leg.

'Isn't there a kinder way of you doing this? Can't you numb my son first?'

'No time for that, hen, we've got a whole ward to collect from. Anyway, he's fine, I've finished now.' She writes your hospital number onto the tube.

'See you next week,' she grins.

*

I slip my hand through the incubator armhole.

'I'm here, Louis, I'm here,' I whisper and your tiny cry settles. I stroke your forehead ever so gently with the tips of my fingers and then lightly run my hand over the knitted wee hat that you're wearing, cradle your head in my palm. Your eyes are tightly shut but I see the tension in your brows lessen. I wait a while until I'm sure your sleep is relaxed then I move my hand and reposition the cotton sheet that's lying crumpled over your middle. I pull it out and down to go over your nappy and legs, cover the splints and intravenous wires still attached. Your tiny feet, deep pink, poke out at the end. Both of your miniature ankles are ringed with a plastic bracelet, one with your name on and the other with your hospital number. I know your number off by heart; I write it every day on the bottles of milk I'm expressing. It's an easy number to remember, you are number 77077 – I like the fact you have a lot of lucky sevens in there.

⁓

The handsome Portuguese doctor enters the lift. He has long eyelashes, warm brown eyes and a toned body beneath those blue operating gowns. I've heard wistful sighs about him from the nurses on the ward; 'Ooo he's so gorgeous,' 'He's a good dancer at the staff party, I'll have you know.' The doctor smiles at us and I smile back and then look away. I'm feeling embarrassed. The last time I saw this doctor he was inspecting me internally. I had passed a large clot of blood after being sent home and it had scared me, it had looked like a brain.

'You fancy him,' Greg says as we step out of the lift.

'What?'

I know he's teasing.

'Come on, who wouldn't? But this is not really the place for that.'

Greg's pulling faces, trying to look like the doctor.

'Stop it.' I'm laughing.

We're heading towards the remote-controlled doors at the entrance of the hospital when a woman with her head down rushes through the doors from outside and nearly bumps into us, stopping abruptly. The woman looks up and shock registers across her face.

'Jessie,' I say in surprise.

'Oh goodness, Alison. I can't believe it, what's happened to you. Who would have thought something like this could possibly happen to someone like you?'

We're all silent as Jessie pauses. 'How's your baby?' she continues in a concerned voice.

'He's doing okay, we hope. He's called Louis. He's moved from intensive care to special care now.'

'Oh, intensive care. I've worked there but it didn't suit me. I couldn't bear hearing a baby cry. I'd go rushing to it. I was always forgetting to wash my hands.'

We're all awkwardly silent. She's trying to smile but her eyes are cast sideways.

'Well, I hope it continues to go well.'

I move aside to let her past.

⌒

The last time I'd seen Jessie was on the day you were born. She'd been summoned by Dr O'Hara to come and explain what was happening. Jessie had looked serious when she came into the small counselling room where I'd been taken and left.

'Oh dear, Alison. You're going to be admitted immediately.'

I was crying in shock.

'Would you like me to call Greg for you?'

'Greg's down in the Borders, he's doing a site survey, there's no way to contact him.'

'Look, I've got your number,' she said kindly, 'I'll leave a message on your answerphone at home. I'll let Greg know where to find you in the ward. Have you got your pregnancy care plan on you?'

I had lifted my handbag onto my lap and pulled the blue booklet out and passed it to her.

'Now let's take you over to the ward.'

⌒

Jessie was my 'main' midwife on the community midwifery Domino scheme. I'd wanted a home birth originally, but because it was my first time they had advised against it. On the Domino scheme I was to be able to go into labour at home, head over to the hospital for delivery and then home again within six hours if all went well. It had seemed like the perfect option.

I'd been enjoying your pregnancy, feeling you growing and kicking inside. People would say, 'Enjoy your last moments of freedom, your life will never be the same again,' and Greg and I would laugh, feel excitement at the thought.

I'd waited all of that previous week to see Jessie before you were born. She had not turned up on Tuesday afternoon as had been arranged so I'd rung her number at the end of the day and left a message on the answerphone. She was apologetic when she called the next morning.

'I'm sorry, Alison, I was waylaid by a delivery.'

'Oh. Jessie, I would like to see you. I'm not feeling so well and I want to check things with you.'

'Now don't you worry; I'm rushing right now but I'll be over tomorrow in the morning. I'll be with you by lunchtime, okay?'

She called again on Thursday lunchtime.

'I'm sorry, I've been delayed again, I'm afraid. It shouldn't take much longer; I'll be with you by the end of the day. In the very unlikely event that I'm not, I'll definitely see you tomorrow.'

She never came.

On Saturday morning I was wondering what to do about being seen. Jessie had told me at our first meeting, 'Alison, for the scheme to work you must follow the Domino rules. We only take on low-risk patients, first pregnancies are not usually allowed, but I've decided you're so healthy you can qualify. The scheme has limited funding so I must stress to you I'm your first point of contact.'

'So I must call you if I have any concerns?'

'Yes, unless it's an emergency. There's no point to the scheme if you keep using the hospital service.'

Jessie had pulled out a pen and ringed her telephone number on the care plan adding her name 'Jessie' beneath.

It was Saturday morning and we were sitting at the kitchen table eating toast.

'What do you think I should do? Do community midwives work at weekends too? Should I try calling again?'

'Who's that?'

Greg had left his toast and gone through the hall to the front door. I could hear laughter as I walked towards it, the daylight spilling down the wooden boards of the floor. Over Greg's shoulder I saw Jessie and someone else, dark haired and slighter, behind her. My heart lifted. *She's come, now I can check.*

'This is my boring case,' Jessie said to the woman with her and then laughed, smiling brightly at me. I'd quietly smiled back as Greg ushered them into the hall. Jessie leaned towards my ear as we walked into the living room.

'I'm sorry to have taken so long in coming and not letting you know. You wouldn't believe the week that I've had.'

They both sat down near the window; Greg offered them a drink.

'No thanks, we want to make this quick. We've been up all night up the road and we're heading home to our beds. I realised you lived here so I thought I'd knock on the off-chance and introduce you to Catriona, too, kill two birds with one stone.'

She turned her head to the left. 'Catriona is one of your six allocated midwives too.'

I was sitting facing them both waiting for Jessie to pause.

'Actually, Jessie, I'm pleased you've come, I'm not feeling too well. I've been wanting to ask you what you think.'

'Okay. Is there something bothering you in particular?'

Catriona said something I didn't catch and Jessie's face broke into a broad grin, her body shaking. I was feeling flushed, my head throbbing at the temples.

'Yes, well, there's a few things. I've not been feeling myself all week. I've got a headache that keeps coming and going and I don't usually get headaches at all.'

'Have you taken any paracetamol?'

'Well, no, I didn't think I could because I'm pregnant?'

'It's okay to take a couple.'

'I had to leave a friend's funeral yesterday and come home to lie down, I felt so tired and fluey. I've been trying to rest but my face still feels puffy and my vision seems to be blurred around the edges of my eyes.'

I lifted my hands up to my face, pressing softly at my temples.

'Oh, that's nothing to worry about. That can happen in pregnancy – your eyesight can change and then it reverts back to normal after.'

'Oh, right. I've been feeling anxious too. The baby doesn't seem to be moving as much as before and my stomach doesn't seem to have grown since I was last checked. I've been looking in my pregnancy book, it says the baby is meant to double in size from twenty-eight to thirty-two weeks and I just don't feel like I've changed at all.'

'Has someone been saying you look small?'

Jessie's voice had hardened.

'Well, yes, actually. I bumped into my friend's mother at the swimming pool on Sunday. I didn't feel well enough to go in, that's not like me either. She said how small I looked.'

'Well, next time someone says something like that to you, I suggest you look them straight in the eye and say, "Oh dear! Do you think something is wrong?"'

My face flushed hot and I felt my eyes welling with tears.

'But I think I'm small too.'

I could hear my voice wavering, my head was beginning to throb again, tears were running down my face.

Jessie had looked across at Catriona again; she glanced back at me and her face turned suddenly serious.

'Let's go into the bedroom and check, eh? I'm sure everything's fine.'

I'd brushed the tears off my cheeks.

I led the way to the bedroom, slipped off my shoes and lay down on the bed. I lifted my blue top and lowered my elasticated trousers to display my rounded belly.

'Let's have a check of that baby.'

Jessie's hands felt my stomach. Catriona bent down, lifting a funnel out of her bag and passed it to Jessie.

'There, that's the head – it's in position already, that's good. Now that means the heart will be around here.'

She pressed her fingers into my side and lifted the funnel-shaped object, placed it beside her fingers and put her ear down to listen.

We were all silent.

I could feel my own heartbeat throbbing in my ears.

One, two, three, four, five, six, seven, eight, nine, ten, eleven, twelve, thirteen, fourteen, fifteen.

'There, I heard it; it's fine, absolutely fine.'

Jessie passed the funnel back to Catriona. My face had broken into a smile.

'That's good,' I said from my prone position, 'but what about the movements? They're reduced and they don't feel like movements or kicks any more but just flutters and only down low like a tickling sensation.'

'Oh, movements change all the time in pregnancy. Are you feeling twelve in a day?'

'Well, yes, just, if a flutter counts?'

'Yes, that's fine then.'

'Ah, we are meant to have taken your blood by now as you're rhesus negative. We'd better do that quickly too.'

I'd not moved. I was still flat on my back and starting to feel uncomfortable.

'Can you put your arm out to your side, Alison? We'll get this blood taken.'

The needle went into my arm but Catriona was talking. She was looking over her shoulder and speaking to Jessie, the needle still in my arm, the syringe half full with blood. Catriona looked back and removed the needle, asked me to put pressure on the puncture.

'There you go. You're fine, we'll be off.'

'See you in two weeks' time.'

Jessie smiled at me lying there as she walked out the bedroom door.

Greg left too. I could hear them all walking through the hall, still laughing, and out of the front door. I heard Greg thanking them, saying he hoped they got some sleep as I struggled to sit up. It felt better being upright; it wasn't comfortable being flat like that. I put my legs over the side of the bed and sat on the edge. I moved along the side and leaned over to pick up my care plan and turned to the back of the booklet. *When are they coming back? What had they meant by two weeks? Were we back to my usual Tuesday?* The return appointments column was blank. *What about my symptoms? Has she put anything about those?* I flicked the book open; that column was blank too. And the blood pressure column, but that wasn't taken, but what's it for? I didn't have a clue. Greg interrupted my train of thought as he entered the bedroom with a wide grin.

'Well, that's a relief then, isn't it; you've got nothing to worry about.'

'I still don't feel too great, though, a headache's started again.'

'Look, you're obviously upset about John's death. Why don't you lie down? I'll pop to the shops and get something nice for lunch.'

⁓

Three months before you were conceived I turned thirty, Greg was thirty-one. On that day I stared at my face in the bathroom mirror and felt a wave of sadness. Life was fun but where were my children? What was I doing at this age having none?

But you were still a surprise of sorts. We'd been planning on travelling around the world. I'd never travelled far but had always craved to. I'd been sensible, studying, working, trying to build a career in landscape architecture, knowing that one day I would want children. *If we don't go now before children we never will*, I had thought. And Greg was convinced he was infertile. No reason why but it was something he had always said to me.

We'd agreed to go for it, go travelling.

'Let's shag around the world,' Greg had said. 'If it's going to happen it may take a while.'

Well, it didn't. It didn't take more than one try.

'That's our plan scuppered,' I'd laughed.

Greg seemed to walk taller that day I told him.

Two days after the midwives' visit, on the eve before you

were born, we'd sat on the sofa playing that favourite game of expectant parents: What shall we call the baby? We were calling out names backwards and forwards.

'Dexter?'

'Rebecca?'

'Baxter?'

'Monty?'

'That's hideous!' Greg had exclaimed. He had an aversion to any name with a public school ring. He liked the idea of a jazz musician in my womb.

'What about Louis?' I said. It had a soft ring but strength to it too. 'It means "fighter", in the book.'

'I quite like that one.'

Who knows what we would have called you if you had been born as you should have been eight weeks later.

You'll need to be a fighter, is what I'd thought the next day.

That night I'd bent over suddenly as I got into bed. A sharp pain stabbed in my belly and I'd bent onto all fours.

'What are you doing?'

'I just got a pain. It's subsiding now.'

'Do you think it's the curry I made for you?'

'I don't know. Greg, I'm still not feeling right and I feel anxious.'

'Why don't you say something at the antenatal class to-morrow?'

'Yes, I was just thinking that. I think I will.'

I lay on the bed and waited to feel you move. You gave me a kick, not a flutter. That made me feel pleased, that was my number twelve. But I'd decided: tomorrow morning I'd go up to the hospital and ask again. I felt a sense of relief. I was sure I was making a fuss about nothing but I couldn't bear the thought of waiting another two weeks to be seen. I'd always felt well so this was unusual. I kept thinking of John – he'd left his mole for too long without going to the doctor. Was I worrying unnecessarily? I didn't want to call Jessie again. I'd decided I'd go against her instructions and double check with someone else at the hospital just to be sure.

That night I had a nightmare. I dreamt of a baby in my arms but the baby didn't look like a baby. It was a child but not a normal-looking child either. It was long, very long and thin – no, scrawny. Its arms hung down from its body and its legs stuck out past my waist. It had reddish hair, and small sharp teeth. I had held it stretched out in my arms away from my body. I could feel its weight and was staring at it horrified. It was looking up at me with a knowing stare. 'Well,' I'd whispered, 'seeing as you can talk what do you want me to call you?' A grating robotic voice had replied, 'Oliver.'

When you were lifted out later that day the doctor had asked, 'So do you have a name?' 'Oliver' screeched through my mind. 'Louis,' I answered. I'm so glad I named you that, I say your name over and over and it always sounds right.

⁓

At the hospital I decided to speak to Dee, the physio running the second part of the antenatal class. The midwife before her had seemed a little bit wet. I'd held back from telling her, thinking she might tell me not to worry and ask when I'd last been seen. Dee, however, seemed efficient; her manner was caring but direct. Her class that week involved breathing techniques during labour. I'd lain on a mat and steadied my breathing, taking deep breaths like she told us to do. I was waiting to feel your first movement that day.

'I'm feeling a little bit worried about my pregnancy.'

'Oh dear, my dear, what's worrying you?'

'Well, I'm worried about my size. My stomach looks small; I don't feel like it's been growing. I look so much smaller than everyone else in the class today.'

Dee looked down at my stomach.

'Yes, you do look small, I agree.'

'And I've not been feeling well recently either. I've been having headaches and my vision seems blurred.'

'Okay dear, have you been seen recently?'

I felt hot. Tears sprang into my eyes again. *This really isn't like me.* I panicked inside; *if I answer 'three days ago' will she still check me?* I didn't answer her question but continued.

'And it's not just that. The movements from the baby feel different, lighter and less frequent. And now I'm starting to feel really anxious because I've not had a movement yet today.'

'When did you last have one?'

'Last night as I was going to bed. I had a pain, a short sharp pain that went away and then I got a kick afterwards, but I've not felt anything since.'

'Wait here. I'm going to go and see if I can arrange for you to have a scan. I'm sure you're fine but let's just put your mind at rest.'

She left me in an empty waiting room beside the scanning room. I helped myself to water from a dispensing machine on my right; I'd been told it was good to drink before a scan. I'd not had a scan since the official one at twelve weeks and I suddenly felt rather buoyant as I waited. *Everything will be absolutely fine and I won't need to worry any more.* Eventually I heard a key in a lock. A nurse had opened the door and motioned me in.

She was very short and had a hunch. Her voice was high and gentle.

'Hello, dear. Just pop yourself up onto the bed. Dee tells me you're feeling a little bit anxious today, not had much movement? Let's have a quick look to check everything is okay.'

The nurse pulled paper sheeting across the bed as she spoke.

She squeezed jelly onto my belly. It was wet and cold.

'Now I'll just run this over your stomach and take a quick look, find the heartbeat. Ah, there it is.'

She moved the rounded probe over and around my belly; at times crosses appeared on the monitor screen as she measured you.

Can I tell if you are a boy or a girl?

'Actually, dear, I'd like you to move across to this other machine over here; it's more detailed. I'm just going to get Dr O'Hara.'

They leaned in together, studying the monitor screen.

'What's that?'

Dr O'Hara paused from the hushed discussion and turned to me. She was petite, slender and seemed terribly astute. She had stridden into the room and straight up to the screen. She was clearly in charge, but her manner was pleasant and she had a soft smile and warm eyes.

'We are just trying to work that out and I need to concentrate, then I will discuss things with you.'

I sat up on the bed and pulled my top back down over my belly, still sticky from the gel.

'We need to keep you in. Your baby is small for its dates; there is the possibility of an abruption, we couldn't be sure. I'm going to instruct that you are given steroids immediately; these will take effect over the next forty-eight hours. We'll get your blood pressure taken and a CTG monitor on you, but the aim will be to deliver within the next twenty-four to forty-eight hours. I'll call for the community midwife, ask her to come and explain things further and take you down to the ward.'

'Shall I go home and get my things?'

She looked startled.

'No, you are being admitted straight away.'

⌇

The needle went into my shoulder.

'That's the steroids done. Now let's get you up on the bed.'

Jelly was placed on my belly again and two patches attached. The monitor started to bleep. The nurse slid a band up my arm and I felt it inflate. Her head was tilted down facing her lap and she was silent. The cuff deflated on my arm and her head shot up and she stared at me.

She was up on her feet.

'I'm just going to find a doctor.'

I was propped up on a hospital bed. I was wearing a hospital gown and it was pulled up to expose my stomach. A light sheet was over me covering my bareness. The ward was quiet. A curtain had been pulled around my cubicle although there was no one next to me on either side. I could hear the comforting bleep of the monitor, your heart, and see the white line as it squiggled across the screen. There was another line crossing it too. *What's that one for?*

The nurse returned with a doctor. This one was tall with

thick brown hair flowing down to her shoulders and an intelligent, serious air. She looked at the monitor, and lifted up the paper trace with the angry lines.

'Have you had bleeding down below?'

'No, I haven't.'

'None at all?'

'No. I had a stabbing pain last night around midnight, lasting around a minute then it went away.'

'What about movements?'

'That's what's been worrying me. They've reduced recently, but I've had none today.'

'I'm sending you straight up to the delivery suite. The trace is concerning and your blood pressure is dangerously high. We need to get it under control, check your bloods. As soon as we can we will deliver you.'

⁓

'When were you last seen?'

'Three days ago.'

The doctor had his back to me. He was muscular and imposing with an arrogant air, but he seemed rather flustered.

'Can you believe it! She was seen three days ago and they did not take her blood pressure.'

He slammed the file down, came over to me, knocked my knees.

'Look, she's hyper-reflexive; she might fit at any moment. Where are the results of those blood tests? Start the emergency protocol now.'

⌣

I have daydreams of what we will do together when you leave hospital. I picture us standing in Kelvingrove Park, the autumn leaves falling around us. I'm holding your hand, the sun is beaming, your blond hair is shining, your red wellington boots are gleaming. You're stamping your feet, up and down, up and down, splashing around in the puddles.

⌣

It is early December and there is sparkling frost on the ground outside. This is a milestone moment, the time you were meant to be born; instead you are eight weeks old and the doctors' round is underway. I pause in the corridor at the top of the ward by the notice board. Two long sections of wall space are dedicated to displaying messages and photographs of babies who've been in this unit. 'Billy sends love to all the doctors and nurses on his third birthday.' And Billy beams out from the photograph with chocolate cake smeared over his face. 'Here's Senga taking her first steps,' says another as a petite red-haired girl steps forward in the photograph. And there are photographs placed next to these ones sent in of them as babies in here. I recognise a couple of the nurses, they look younger, smiling out towards the camera, the parents beside them, the baby clothed and wrapped up ready to go home.

My heart rises as I dream of the day that I'll send in your picture. I imagine the day we leave, carrying you out of this hospital unit for good, waving goodbye to the nurses as the camera snaps. I picture taking your photograph aged three, a boy with golden curls like my brother and a cheeky grin. You're bombing about on your trike, whizzing around the trees in the park, scaring those squirrels. And I picture myself sitting down at my desk to write my letter of thanks, taking you down the road to the post box, lifting you up to drop the letter in.

I steel myself, look across to the memoriam board. It also has photos but only of babies, cards of remembrance, poems. All dreams have been shattered. *That little one didn't make it.* My heart constricts. He lasted so long. He looks a little like you.

I see the doctors leaving the ward. I move away from the notice board and head down the corridor past the main intensive care room. I glance through the glass wall towards the row of incubators where you lay a few weeks ago. Some of the little ones move their arms in the air as if in a womb, as if they are floating. I find it mesmerising to see, although I don't stop and stare. *Remember the rules*: you must look only at your own baby.

Your arms floated briefly when your arm splints were

51

removed, the ventilator gone. They lifted up into the air and moved in a slow-motion wave. Today when I reach you, you've tucked your hand under your head and have a contented look as you sleep. You are starting to look like you're not in a womb any more. Today you look like a baby, a special baby-unit baby.

All of the babies in here have a certain look. Their heads elongated, their faces and foreheads long and thin; the soft bones of their skull squashed by the weight of their brains as they lie positioned sideways in their incubators. The nurses change your position a number of times each day but you still have the look, and Ludo has it too. Ludo lies opposite in his own special room. The rooms are small glass boxes, big enough to hold an incubator and a chair. Both of your lids are off now, they've become beds that hold you as you grow. You have a virus. You've caught it in the hospital somehow but it doesn't seem to be affecting you. The doctors aren't worried but they don't want it to spread, not to the more vulnerable ones in here.

I don't know why Ludo is in his room. You've been in here a week now and I've begun to smile at Ludo's mother. We acknowledge each other, neither of us asking any questions, though. Ludo's room has an abundance of soft toys positioned around his bed and well-wishing cards stuck to the glass walls of his room. Today his room looks different. Today there are lots of balloons and both parents sit by his side.

Three of the main nurses have appeared outside Ludo's room; one holds something in her hand.

'A hundred days old today, Ludo.'

You are forty days behind.

'Here is your special certificate.'

'Ludo is now an honorary member of our especially special hundred club.'

Ludo lies with his eyes closed. He has a calm look on his squashed face as if he has peaceful dreams.

One week later, Ludo's room is empty. No parents, no cards, no teddies, no incubator. There was no warning.

'Where's Ludo gone – has he moved rooms?'

The nurse looks sad.

'He's at rest, poor wee thing. Unfortunately, there are some in here that we just know won't ever be going home.'

⌒

Dr Nook rushes down the corridor. He's always rushing by. He spots me and stops.[

'Ah, just to say we've got the genetic tests back. They have come back as normal – his chromosomes are complete. He's a normal boy, just as I thought.'

⌒

It is mid-December and Dr Thompson is listening to your heart.

'Nope, not a sound. I think I can safely say it has closed.'

53

His face breaks into a wide grin, his crescent-shaped eyes have a twinkle.

'Some of the younger doctors in here call me old-fashioned but it just shows that sometimes patience and waiting can be the best way, especially given the odds we were faced with for Louis.'

He places the stethoscope into the large pocket of his white coat.

'Now that the valve has closed Louis should make much quicker progress. We can now increase his feeds, get some weight on him, work towards you taking him home.'

My heart soars. This is the first time that home has been mentioned.

'It would be preferable if we could get Louis off the oxygen before that happens; he's become dependent – this can happen. Sometimes it can take a long time before they are ready to cope without it and if this is so we have to send them home still using it. You'll need training, equipment and bottles. I'll arrange for you to be shown what it entails.'

I've been watching your oxygen levels for weeks before this latest news. A probe is touching your toe, held there with Velcro. Its rounded glass glows red and your toe does too. Occasionally it comes loose when you move and needs to be repositioned back onto your toe.

'It really needs to be at least ninety-five per cent, a hundred per cent is what we are after.'

A clear plastic tube with two prongs runs into your nose.

The tube wraps around both sides of your face and is held there with tape. The two ends wrap together behind your head and lead away out of the incubator to the oxygen tank.

I've watched the nurses checking the monitor, tweaking the levels flowing down your nose, writing it on the clip board. Sometimes they are able to reduce the quantity of oxygen, turn the dial to allow a little bit less when you've reached the magic hundred on the machine and then sometimes they need to add a little bit more when you dip below ninety-five. An alarm triggers immediately whenever it dips below ninety. Then a nurse appears quickly, checks and increases the flow, waits to see you stabilise. The alarm has been triggering less and less as the weeks have gone by. Now it hardly comes on at all. You are stable, hovering on ninety-five on a very low flow.

'He's nearly there, I'll try again.'

Susan lowers the level down to a trickle. You must panic. Your numbers drop and she turns it back up again. The skin-to-skin contact is helping. Whenever I can I lift you and lie you belly down onto my bare chest, feel the shared warmth of our skins, and your levels rise instantly up to a hundred and the nurse passing by tries again to reduce the oxygen bit by bit.

⁓

It's Christmas Day and we're a little bit later than usual. We want to spend Christmas Day with you. Susan greets us, she must have drawn the short straw but she's beaming.

'Your wee Louis, he's come off the oxygen this morning. He's taken us all by surprise.'

Hey Louis, is that your present for us?

Dr Thompson has popped into the ward just to check on things. He can't keep away.

'This is really good news. Now that Louis is off the oxygen the thing that prevents him from being able to go home is the need to be able to feed independently. I think it will need to be bottle. You could try breast first if you wish? I know that the midwives are keen to promote this but to be honest we've not had much success with that in here.'

'Yes, I would like to try if I can.'

'I thought you might say that. You've done well to express for so long. I'll book the Mother and Baby room and ask the breast-feeding nurse to come and see you. I suggest you come in tomorrow for a few days and nights, see how you get on.'

We are going to be alone together for the first time.

After Dr Thompson leaves us, I wait by your incubator for the breast-feeding nurse to arrive. A tube still runs down your throat. Every four hours a nurse comes to feed you, squirts 100 millilitres of my milk mixed with formula into your stomach. I've been told that the formula will help you to put on weight.

The breast-feeding nurse appears. She still has those pink moist lips, deathly white hands. I haven't seen her since she sent me home with the milking machine. I shudder.

'Shall we try and establish breast-feeding for Louis? It's really the best thing for him and you've done so well expressing, it would be a shame for you not to continue.'

I don't need any convincing. I've been dreaming of this all along.

'It's important you master latching on. Don't let him try a bottle. Once he's had one of those in his mouth it's unlikely he'll breast-feed. Bottles are easier to feed from, you see. It's a different mouth movement entirely.'

The next day I carry you up the corridor. It feels strange to be able to carry you freely in my arms. Nurses offer encouraging comments. We walk past the intensive care unit, the notice board, the doors to outside. I walk on further; I've not been up here. Our room is up near the doctors' consulting rooms. The room has a window. *Maybe we can have some fresh air?* It looks over the car park, past clumps of trees and out over the city. There is a bed for me and an open incubator bed for you. All monitors are gone, no bleeping, no sounds of alarms; the room is uncannily quiet. A tube still runs down your throat for feeding if this fails. The milking machine sits on a table and the bottle steriliser sits there too. And then there's a chair.

You are dressed in a tiny sea blue towelling babygro, the door is closed and I'm sitting in the chair and trying to latch you on gently.

'No, no, that won't do, it will never work like that.'

She tickles your cheek and you open your mouth. I see the feeding tube running beneath the roof of your mouth, disappearing into darkness at the back of your throat. Her hand cups the back of your head and she shoves your mouth onto my breast, holds you firmly in place. Your jaw moves once then stops.

'That didn't work. Let's try again.'

Milk is leaking from my nipple, dripping all over my top, soaking into your sleep suit.

An hour has passed.

An hour of this nurse shoving you onto me, one jaw movement then two at the most and then nothing. You act as if you are comatose. As soon as you feel milk trickle into your stomach you stop. You just completely stop still. Your arms drop down to your side and you appear to wait for your stomach to fill.

'Let's try again with the next feed,' the nurse says. 'You'd better express now. Use the syringe, feed that into your wee one. I'll be back again in a couple of hours to try again.'

I lie you down and go onto the machine, pump out what's left of my milk, feed it to you down the tube. I wind you, change your nappy, sterilise the pumping equipment.

The nurse returns: she is keen to succeed.

'If we keep persevering it will come in the end.'

'That's it, you're getting him to latch on there.'

'Don't worry. Express and feed him. We'll try again.'

I'm exhausted.

This has gone way beyond anything I could have imagined and my breasts hurt like hell. After three days and nights the nurse suggests that I go home, get some sleep and come back again for another go.

'Is it not impossible?'

'You're just overtired right now.'

I return and try again. I try and I try. When the nurse's shift ends and darkness falls I lie on the bed and cry.

I cannot do this any longer.

The pregnancy book is open by my bed, the hospital literature too. It tells me I just have to keep persevering; it will come in the end.

I give up.

I stop pumping and my breasts swell.

Engorge.

And it is agony. I lie miserable in our bath at home and see my milk, your milk, swirl like white smoke into the water; I feel the warmth of the water lessen the pain.

On the third day the swelling reduces, by the fourth the milk is gone and I feel an enormous sense of relief. *It is over.* There was nothing more I could have done. I feel optimistic for us now we're onto the next stage. Now it is bottles, and you've already taken to them well.

I'm at home getting ready to come and see you. The milking machine is gone from our bedroom. It felt good to say goodbye to that monster. I'm sleeping through the night. That's better too; I'll get my strength up before you come home. There's a knocking sound on our door. I haven't opened the door in a long while but Greg is out.

There's a woman standing on our doorstep. I recognise her, *where from?* I know: her name is Hazel, a fellow artist, but I barely know her. I'd met her once in the kitchen of a friend's house; I'd found her angry and somewhat intense. She'd graphically described her home birth to me. *Was I pregnant then?* How she'd given birth in the corner of her living room, had snarled at the midwives to keep away as the baby came out. What's she doing here?

'Hello?'

I don't invite her in.

'I heard that your milk has gone.'

How the hell does she know that?

'I know a way to get it back.'

'No thanks; I've let it go. Louis wasn't able to feed from me.'

She ignores what I say and instead she elaborates, explaining about an amazing NCT woman who knows how to get breast milk to come back. She's breathless and animated, her rosy face flushed. From what she is saying this woman could draw milk from a stone.

This isn't the first time and it won't be the last that I am preached at, told about all of the things I should and could have done, things I can still do for you. All the miracles that could happen if I had just believed, had just tried a little bit harder.

'Go away, will you?'

We are having a trial run. It is New Year's Day and the doctors have said that we can take you home for twelve hours.

It's nine in the morning and I'm carrying you out of the hospital in my arms. Your eyes are closed but I sense you are not sleeping. I sense you can feel the cold air on your cheeks. I place your tiny body into a car seat facing backwards in the back of the car and I sit next to you as Greg drives us home.

We are so excited.

You keep your eyes tightly shut and are very still. Every so often I place my finger under your nose just to check you are breathing and I feel your breath lightly brush my skin.

I chatter to you, we both do.

'This is it, Louis, nearly home.'

'Here we are, up the steps and in here.'

It's quiet outside. I can tell the flats all around are empty, that people are away visiting relatives or asleep recovering from celebrating all night.

And we will be celebrating with you today.

Greg unlocks the front door and I carry you in in your car seat. I lift you out and lie you on the sheepskin rug on the bed. I've been taking this into hospital so you should know it. It had helped your oxygen levels rise too. I'm convinced it helps you to feel safe lying in the warmth of the wool.

Your eyes are still closed but I know you're not sleeping; your body is tense. I pick you up and hold you in my arms, walk you around the flat, pass you to Greg to hold.

Your eyes remain shut all day.

I've fed you three bottles with your eyes closed, and still they are closed. You are as still as can be.

Is there something wrong?

You've never behaved like this before. You've always taken a peek at us, opened your eyes, looked around.

'I can't take this any longer.'

'Neither can I.'

We get back in the car and take you back to the hospital three hours early. As we enter the ward I feel the heat, hear the bleeps down the corridor and I see your eyes open a crack. You are back.

This is it. It is ninety-nine days since you were born and we are finally taking you home. I have dressed you in a padded blue coat and a fleecy blue hat and gently placed you into the car seat. Your eyes are closed but I'm ready for that now.

Karen appears with a camera. 'Let's have one for the notice board.'

Greg and I crouch down beside you smiling and other nurses appear to say their goodbyes.

'Are you sure you don't want to stay for one more day, Louis?' Susan calls out. 'You'll miss getting your certificate!'

'I think that we'll do without,' I say laughing, my stomach clenching as Ludo's face flashes into my mind. I have to block that memory. You have made it onto the wall. My dream is coming true.

The discharging nurse steps forward as we head towards the exit door. She is older than most of the nurses and has a motherly air.

'Now my dears, remember you must treat him just like any other baby.'

'Really?'

'Yes. Take him home and forget all about this.'

Can I really breathe again?

Dr Nook's head pops out of his room as we pass.

'Just one thing before you leave us that I meant to mention: there's my follow-up clinic I run for all of the babies in here. You'll be getting a letter in the post. We'd like you to come back up now and then, just to check that all's going okay. I'll see you in two weeks' time I should think.'

~

You keep your eyes closed for a full three days. I know to expect it now. You must be overwhelmed by the sudden change in temperature, the disappearance of all those sounds, the appearance of new ones. You are like marble. Your chest doesn't move. Your breathing is so shallow that it's invisible to my eye and I check with my finger under your nose again as I carry you around in my arms.

You play dead very well but I don't panic this time: I wait. And then I notice the skin on your eyelids smoothing, your eyebrows losing their furrow. I see two tiny black slits appearing ever so slightly, peeping. You move your head, just a little, from side to side, and then on day four you open your eyes, you open them wide.

⌒

I carry you in my arms up in the lift, press the buzzer and turn right away from the ward. It is like that world doesn't exist to us now you are home. I don't see any of the nurses, busy elsewhere with other wee ones who've come in and replaced you.

Our hospital letter invited us to attend the Monday clinic. I've just discovered from the nurse at reception that there are two clinics each week. Monday clinic is for babies expected to catch up and Tuesday clinic is for those who already clearly will not. This in itself is a milestone for us. The fact that you are here on a Monday gives us reassurance that all will be fine.

I recall Dr Thompson's reassuring talk with us in those early days when you were just born. Your ultrasound scans – how promising they were; how unusual it was for babies in here to not even have a minor bleed on the brain.

'You know, only five per cent of babies in here get no bleeds at all and Louis is one of those. It is extremely promising for you.'

I sit holding you in the small waiting room with other parents. There is a row of chairs along two of the walls and toys piled up in a box on the floor in a corner; some are scattered about, as a baby crawls and a toddler totters around them. I look at this baby and infant and I picture you in a few months' time sitting there, banging that rattle, putting it into your mouth.

We are called through and Dr Nook takes your measurements and plots your growth on a chart. He uses your expected due date in December, *my birthday*, as zero, calls it your corrected date, the day you should have been born.

'It's expected for there to be slight delay at first, which is why we correct the age. By the time Louis is two he should have caught up with his peers.'

You were eight weeks early, not that early for a lot of the babies in here, but early all the same. The statistical outcome for a 'thirty-two weeker' is extremely good. But you are slightly different. You'd been starved in my womb and the problem had gone undetected until Dee had got me that scan. You weighed 920 grams when you were born, less than a bag of sugar, and closer in weight to a twenty-seven-week-old baby, although we are told it's your gestational age that counts for your well-being.

'We'd have got your baby out sooner than this if we could, if we'd known,' I remember Dr Hamilton telling me as he'd paced the room waiting for my blood pressure to lower, waiting for the blood clotting results; he had to check I wouldn't bleed to death before getting you out.

Dr Nook explains that taking regular measurements and plotting them onto the growth chart will help him to check your progress. Your plotted dot sits just beneath the third centile, the final line. If you fall much further you'll fall off.

'It's to be expected right now,' he explains. 'Louis was born starved, and he had to be starved in here for a while too for the ductus to close. Hopefully he'll make his way up the chart or at least keep a steady progress along where he is now.'

He pauses then continues. He is speaking as if it's an aside, with no apparent concern that it is going to apply to you.

'It's the tailing off we need to be on the alert for. That is often the first sign for us doctors to look out for as it can indicate possible future problems.'

You've woken on my lap and smile when the doctor coos at you, jump in my arms when the doctors claps behind your ear.

He's pleased with your progress today.

'He's coming on nicely: meeting his milestones, putting on weight. I'll arrange to see you again in four weeks' time.'

⁓

It's the end of January and I have our baby routine underway; it still feels stunning not to go up to the hospital every day. In comparison all is quiet and still and a little bit cold. The hospital was hot; I would need to strip down to a t-shirt, but now instead I can breathe cool air with you here in our flat. My heart has settled, my throat has loosened and I can gently hum into your ear.

Greg has gone off to work, he goes every morning, and I wander around our small flat. I walk between each of the rooms with you swaddled in a blanket and resting on my shoulder. As I walk I gently pat your nappied bottom and rub your back.

I move into the living room and then the spare bedroom at the front of the house. These rooms are my least favourite, I feel overlooked by the black windows of the red sandstone tenements opposite. I walk down the internal t-shaped hallway stepping on colours on the floorboards, spilled from the light through the stained-glass window in the main front door. I go into our bright yellow kitchen and up to the white sash window that overlooks our wintery garden. I turn on the kettle, pour boiling water into a Pyrex jar and place a bottle of formula milk into it to warm, then I go back out with you still on my shoulder and into our bedroom (you sleep here now in the carrycot beside us). I sit down on the edge of the bed and lift you off my shoulder, around and down and nestle you into the crook of my arm, and I tilt the bottle, let the teat touch your lips and you open your mouth expectantly.

You gulp down the milk.

I hear the sound of whole bubbles of air as you swallow; hear the strange bumping sound as it travels down your chest. I've learnt to stop feeding you straight away when this happens. I stop. I lift you over my shoulder, pat your back, rub my hand up and down until you burp and vomit a little on the muslin cloth. And then I continue to feed you.

It's starting to take longer and longer each time this happens and your vomiting is increasing by the week and you seem to be developing colic. I've noticed you're pulling your legs up like a frog to your rib cage, and you cry and you cry and you cry.

Your head and your length are continuing along the third centile line of the graph but today your weight has dipped. It's a different doctor, not Dr Nook. I explain that you've been struggling with your feeds.

'Yes, it might just be that.'

'Are you worried?'

'Well, it is hard to tell right now.'

'What do you mean?'

'Well, we just have to wait and see but I'd like you to come back in two weeks this time, keep a closer eye. I'd like the physio to take a quick look at Louis too. Can you wait in the waiting room again for a moment?'

We are called through again and there is Zoe, the physio from the ward. She takes you from my arms and places you on a mat on the floor. She lays you onto your stomach and you start to cry. Doesn't she know about your pigeon chest? That must hurt you. Your rib cage is pointed as a result of the ventilator pumping against your bones. I try to tell her but she's busy rolling you onto your side, your other side and now back again onto your front. She's trying to get you to lift your head up as you lie on your chest. You are crying harder, screaming now. She hands you back to me with a serious nod. I'm trying to comfort you, calm you down. The doctor and physio are speaking quietly together, something about tone, posterior, your head.

We leave the clinic feeling worried, Greg and I. I have a gnawing feeling in my stomach, a twist in my heart as we meet Dr Thompson in the corridor. He holds his hand above your head, wiggles his fingers and then moves his index finger from side to side. You are following with your eyes, keeping up with his finger, and then you break into a smile. A big, bright, wide smile.

'There's nothing wrong with this one.'

Dr Thompson looks pleased. He strides off with a grin on his face and my heart lifts again.

We decide to go on a holiday.

'Let's try and recover from everything that's happened in the last six months; do what the nurse told us, forget about the hospital.'

We choose a pretty stone cottage painted white in the heart of the Cairngorms; it is nestled beneath hills in a forested glen. We joke together as we set off; we call this holiday our honeymoon.

The cottage is situated on the edge of a hamlet and its

back garden has a monkey puzzle tree and a leaning Scots pine. The garden backs onto a conifer wood and I notice there are deer tracks pressed into the soft moss ground when I open the back door early this morning. At the front of the house is a small footpath that winds its way up to the left and around a pretty marsh pond and then the path winds down again along the other side of the water's edge. This pond with a backdrop of silver birch trees is our view from the cottage's kitchen window and on this bright March morning it is showing the first signs of spring in its reeds.

Earlier this morning the sun had streamed in through our bedroom window and Greg and I had smiled at each other at our good fortune with the weather. *It is beautiful and peaceful here; maybe at last we will start to recover.*

Now Greg has gone for a walk through the woods and I am sitting on a chair in the kitchen with you on my lap. I've spread a large plastic sheet across the kitchen floor in case you vomit after I've fed you. To my horror you vomit more than I've ever seen you vomit before. I try feeding you again. I warm the milk, hold you in the crook of my arm, place the bottle to your lips. You are hungry. You keep your eyes closed and drink big gulps. I hear you swallow air and instantly stop, tilt you forwards with your chin cupped in my hand, and as I pat your back you vomit again. Everything. It splatters across the sheet. *Thank goodness I brought this with me.*

I wonder what to do as I comfort you writhing in my arms. My chair is facing the kitchen window and I stare out of it feeling anxious. I try feeding you one more time and you vomit again violently, so I find the number in the visitor book and pick up the telephone on the sideboard and call the local doctor. I arrange to be seen at his surgery in the next village this afternoon.

The doctor is bad tempered and short with me.

'All babies vomit.'

'But he's vomiting everything.'

'Oh, it can look like that but it won't be so. He will be getting what he needs. He looks fine. Take him home.'

We go back to the holiday home. You vomit your next feed and your next. You seem hot; your breathing is laboured.

I barely dare to go to sleep that night in case you vomit in your sleep. I lay your pram bed next to our bed and lie looking down at you through the night.

We are exhausted and worried. We are always exhausted and worried these days. Is this any different?

The next day I sit in the kitchen feeding you and vomit spurts onto the floor again. I get down on the floor, get out my plastic syringe and suck up all the vomit. I squirt it back into the hundred-millilitre bottle: ninety-five millilitres.

By the evening Greg and I are arguing with each other in desperation. At eleven I call Len.

'Look at Louis's chest. How is he breathing?'

I open your babygro to look. Your breathing is laboured. Your chest pulls right in and up under your rib cage.

'I don't care if you have to get that doctor out of bed, he has to look at Louis again.'

71

I call the doctor. He sounds grumpy, sighing when I tell him my uncle's a doctor and is insisting that he sees you.

'Come down to the surgery,' he says.

The doctor is standing outside when we arrive. He looks at you and calls an ambulance.

'You need to be taken to Inverness hospital.'

You are wrapped in a blanket in my arms. The door of the ambulance closes and the doctor disappears from my view. I notice from this angle his coat is covering his pyjamas, poking out at the bottom. His face has a worn expression. I suppose it is one in the morning now.

The oxygen mask is over your face and your chest still pulls sharply under your ribs. I feel the movement of the vehicle and I hold you tight. I suddenly realise the ambulance man is talking to me.

'How old is your son?'

'Six months,' I whisper, say nothing more.

'Ah, so is my son; he's six months and massive. Will eat anything you put in front of him. He sits there banging his spoon wanting more and more . . .'

The doctors are worried. They think you have meningitis.

You need a lumbar puncture. I'm asked to leave the room. I feel uncertain. *Should I leave?*

'Is it right to leave?'

'It is for the best.'

'Really, is it right to leave my baby?'

'Yes, or they associate the pain that they experience with you.'

I feel confused about this. Should I leave you all alone when you are to have things done to you?

I hear your scream.

You scream an agonising, terrified, desperate scream. I feel sick to the bone. The door opens. The doctor's face is blanched.

'It didn't work. He fought me off. I've never known any baby react like that.'

I hold you tight. I vow I will never ever leave you like that again.

The nurses find us amusing. We are known as the honeymoon couple spending it in Inverness hospital. They are kind and concerned for you lying naked in an incubator in an oxygen tent. You're on a drip for dehydration and have an infection but the meningitis scare is over.

This morning a new nurse has arrived with a suction tube in her hand. She sticks it down your nose and explains she is sucking up mucus out of your stomach. Her face has a look of intense enjoyment as she performs the task. As she finishes she turns her head towards me.

'Look at him. That's an apology, that is!'

She walks away shaking her head, laughing to herself. What does she mean? Then I realise she was pointing at your penis. I'd like to punch that nurse. I don't but when I see her my anger boils.

⌒

It's a custom in Glasgow to throw money into a pram or a pushchair if you see a new baby go by. People slow their pace to look at you, to check you out. You are so tiny but you don't look like an innocent baby: you look like a little old man.

'How can that be?' you can tell they are thinking, turning their heads, nudging their partners.

And some that wander the streets speedily in pairs, with legs you could snap and straggled hair, suddenly stop, turn and stare.

'Hey, look at that.'

'Where?'

'There. Over there.'

'It's a fella!'

'A fella?'

'Yes, that's a wee fella.'

'Hey, you've got a wee fella in there.'

The next clinic visit shows you are still losing weight.

'The chart shows that Louis's head and body are keeping in line with the centile but his weight is continuing to fall. We need to keep a close eye.'

'What does this mean?'

'We're not sure right now. He's failing to thrive. He might catch up again when we have tackled all his reflux and feeding problems. We're uncertain how much this is impacting on his development. We will just have to wait and see.'

'Are you worried about Louis?'

'Your son will go to a normal school, that's all I can say.'

ONE

You are still tiny. You have startled blue eyes, a peaky face and spiky wispy blond hair. You curl up your fingers and smile brightly at me as I coo and then sometimes you look a bit puzzled. You are perfect in my eyes even though we have worries.

You are one year old and your weight has not caught up yet. You weigh 5.9 kilograms, that's half the weight of an average child your age. I dress you each morning and my favourite outfit is a soft pair of tartan blue and yellow trousers, and a sweet little jumper knitted especially for you by my cousin Anna. And I carry you everywhere. I've bought a baby papoose that straps easily around my waist and you snuggle down in a hump on my chest, or else I hitch you around my waist. You are happy in these positions most of the time, being warm and close to me, looking around, and it means I can do practical chores with you held there, in between all of the drawn-out feeding.

～

I've arranged to meet Greg at twelve to walk back to our flat together. He's taken you for a walk around Kelvingrove Park while I've come here to Waterstones on Sauchiehall Street to do some research. I've wanted to do this for a while but it has been difficult to find a time when I can be away from you for long. I want to know exactly what pre-eclampsia is. I've heard the word used by the doctors. I've been told I had it. But I don't understand what it actually is. I realise it has something to do with my blood pressure being dangerously high, but nothing more. What is it? What causes it? I want to know because I want to try for another baby; I want to know if it could happen again.

I can't find anything in my general pregnancy book at home or on the shelves downstairs in the bookshop under 'Mother and Baby' so I climb the stairs to the third floor and look around for 'Obstetrics'; I find it within the Medical section. I start looking through the maternal medicine books and I find one entitled *Myles Textbook for Midwives*. I open it and find a section called 'Pre-eclampsia and hypertension in pregnancy'. It discusses how pre-eclampsia is one of the most common and serious complications in pregnancy, that it is one of the main conditions that a midwife should be looking out for when conducting an antenatal check. It states that pre-eclampsia is a combination of high blood pressure over 140/90 and one plus of protein in the urine. This is why a midwife should always check both the blood pressure and urine on each visit.

I'm frozen in my seat.

The book lists further symptoms for the mother: oedema – the sudden swelling of the feet, ankles, face and hands; severe headaches; visual problems such as blurred vision and flashing lights; pain just below the ribs; feeling very unwell. And the main signs in the foetus are not growing so well and reduced movements.

I'm stunned.

I hadn't appreciated until this moment that I had been suffering from almost all of the main symptoms of pre-ec-lampsia.

It's coming up to twelve so I leave the bookshop and walk along the main street away from the city centre, cross over the busy bypass by bridge and cut down a side street to reach the gate at the edge of the park near a terrace of of-fices. There's Greg standing waiting by the entrance while you are lying back in the three-wheeler pushchair with your eyes closed. You are dressed in an all-in-one snow-suit and nestled into the sheepskin rug that we've taken to putting in the pushchair's base, and over your body there's a blanket.

Greg looks pleased to see me.

'Hey, you wouldn't believe who I met in the park with Louis.'

'No, tell me, who?'

'Remember that Alsatian that I told you about? The one that shot into the road in front of the car with no warning, when I was on the way to see you and Louis up at the hospital? When the police were called? I was convinced it had died; it was bleeding all over the road. Well, we turned the corner by the pond and I saw it, the Alsatian. I couldn't believe it. I rushed up to the owner. "Hey do you remember me? I'm the man who knocked over your dog this time last year. It's alive, that's great to see." But the woman didn't look pleased, she just pulled its lead and walked away.'

'Greg, are you kidding me? She's not going to have been happy to be reminded of that by you.'

And poor Greg looks puzzled; he can't understand why. When Greg first told me about the Alsatian I was still in deep trauma; it barely registered then, but I realise now how awful that must have been for him, both of those incidents together. His joyful reaction today is to turn these events into happy endings, and they are, but for the dog owner the memory of what happened is still traumatic. The Alsatian's alive and we are out here in the park, us three, as a family. The journey so far has not been smooth sailing but we are hopeful it will all start getting easier.

⁓

Janet – Greg's mother, your grandmother – has come to visit. You're fourteen months old now and this is the first time she has met you. She looks at you in your bouncing chair. She stares down at you from her seat in the kitchen; down at you in your blue canvas chair on the floor.

'There's something not quite right about him. He's not like any baby I've come across before.'

Janet has had four babies of her own so she should know. But she's become an alcoholic so I try not to take any notice of what she says as she gazes at you.

⁓

The taxi stops at the lights, we are heading to the hospital for another of those fortnightly clinic visits. We've been making this trip for over a year now. The cab driver hasn't stopped talking since we got in.

'As long as they're okay, that's what matters. It doesn't matter what sex they are and all of that nonsense, as long as they're okay that's the main thing.'

But what if they're not?

'My brother, now he was born early you know – only a pound he was too. You should see him now, he's six foot and there's absolutely nothing wrong with him.'

People keep telling me a similar story. So many that I've checked with the doctors.

'Doctor, do you mind my asking – can a one pound baby survive?'

'No. Not that light. There are those that weigh a little bit more who may survive. It's the gestation that matters. Twenty-three weeks is the earliest and those will most likely face serious disabilities if they do.'

I stay silent in the taxi.

You can't stand, you can't crawl, and you can't sit up unaided. You can't roll over; you find it difficult to lift your head. You are fifteen months old and we are heading up in the lift to the clinic again. I've decided to be direct. I can feel the swelling in my belly – you are going to have a little brother or sister. No one knows about it yet, I've not reached twelve weeks, but it is suddenly dawning on me that things are not improving with you: things are getting worse week by week.

'Dr Nook, does my son have cerebral palsy?'

'I don't find that a helpful term.'

'Well, does he have it or not?'

'It is now apparent that Louis will have some movement difficulties. How mild or severe is difficult to tell right now. We'll just have to wait and see.'

You are always crying, always agitated, writhing around, but it is hardly surprising as you are covered in eczema. Like lichen on a stone, it has spread across your forehead, over your torso and encased the creases in your arms and legs. No wonder you are in a constant state of agitation and distress. I lie close to you on the bed and try to distract you by stroking your body ever so lightly, massaging your scalp so that you enter a trance, find release in sleep.

We wait a relentlessly long time in the hospital waiting room to see the dermatologist, Dr Lyme. You get distressed as we sit here and I wonder if it's your skin getting agitated by the heat in this airless building.

We are wet bandaging you at the moment. Plastering you in ointment and wrapping your limbs in Tubifast bandages. We are limiting your diet too. We've realised you are allergic to some foods. At first the doctors were dismissive as it is apparently rare, but you are. We've discovered you're allergic to all sorts of things: nuts and peas, fish and lentils, sesame and chocolate too. The doctors have become so concerned about your lack of weight gain that you were admitted to hospital again last month and tube fed to see if that could help. I'd slept by your side on a hospital chair. I'm seven months pregnant now. *What is going to happen when the new baby comes?*

It didn't work. The tube threaded down your throat and into your stomach incensed you. The nurse would ask me to hold your hands, your arms but as soon as I let go you pulled the tube out, gagging as it came up your throat. I'd try to distract you but it was impossible. You screamed so hard for so long that the doctors aborted the plan and sent us home after a day and a night. Now they are suggesting a gastrostomy, they see it as a last resort. You are booked in for surgery in a few months' time. I'm concerned. How will this work? You will rip at a tube if it's fitted into your stomach, cause a wound, an infection that could become serious. We are trying to find any possible way to prevent this operation having to go ahead.

I am waiting to have your diet and weight assessed at the dermatology clinic; we've been in the waiting room for over an hour. Dr Lyme's clinic is running late. It always runs late. The waiting room contains a row of moulded plastic seats fixed in a line to the floor. The air is stagnant and hot. A television is suspended from the wall and CBeebies is on. There is a play den and musical toys. Children and toddlers run in and out, opening and shutting the play door, interacting with each other. You can't and you are frustrated. The fluorescent lights shine harshly down on us. *How much longer?* A nurse steps forward and calls out a name that is not yours.

This appointment is important. The doctors are monitoring your weight loss carefully. It will determine when you will have to have the gastrostomy operation. You won't drink any more. Not at all. As soon as you could take solids you refused. Now we have to get all your fluid into you through your food. It has to be pureed and runny; you don't seem to be able to chew. Later I will find out that this is part of your cerebral palsy condition but right now I don't know this. I've been cooking, pureeing, blending, fresh meat and vegetables and fruit, but you prefer to eat custard. You keep your mouth closed, clam it shut as I try to persuade you to open your mouth. I place plastic spoons under your nose heaped with freshly pureed fruit and veg but you wriggle from side to side in your high chair and refuse to eat it. Last week I gave up on my homemade cooking and I brought every single flavour of tined baby food from the Co-op desperate to get something into you. You wouldn't eat any of the flavours except the very last tin, the tin of egg custard. You opened your mouth so wide and gulped it down, it was all gone in an instant and you gestured for more. Now that you've tasted egg custard it is all that you want to eat; feeding you nutritious food has become a challenge every day.

And there's also your eczema to contend with. We will try anything that might help improve it. I tried homeopathy first. I have friends who swear by its miraculous results and I wanted to believe: I need miracles to happen. I put you through six months of visits and pills and your eczema got steadily worse while the homeopath told me that it had to before it could get better. When he told me your eczema was an angry trauma resulting from Greg not being present at your birth, I snapped. What a thing to choose given all the things that have happened. *Oh fuck off, will you?*

The Chinese doctor has been better. We went to see him four weeks ago, having heard that Chinese medicine can be successful with eczema. We went to a tiny shop down on Dumbarton Road. There in the window were rows of glass jars containing dried roots, bark and other indecipherable things. They were displayed on shelves behind the counter too. I held you in my arms as the fatherly Chinese man looked at your eyes, your eyelids, your tongue, your skin. As he took your pulse he seemed concerned, his jovial face became serious.

'I think we should forget about the eczema right now. It is more important that he gets fluid into him.'

He looked down at me.

'You are pregnant?' His voice sounded surprised. 'This is not good, you should only have one baby. This baby needs your undivided attention.'

This Chinese man was voicing my fears out loud. What have I done bringing another child into this world with you? How will I be able to cope, give it happiness too?

'But wait,' the man added. 'When is your baby due?'

'Late August.'

'Ah, okay, yes, this is good after all. Your child Louis is born in the year of the rat. Your new baby will be born in the year of the tiger. The tiger carries the rat on its back. This is good, it all makes sense, this will be what he needs.'

We were sent away with a mixture of roots and leaves to boil in water for four hours. We were told to do this every day for the next four weeks and then to come back and see him again.

'Louis doesn't drink,' I tried to tell him but he didn't seem to hear.

I boiled the concoction until it reduced to a black syrupy liquid to the quantity of a test tube and I dribbled it into your mouth.

And it made the house stink.

Your name is called eventually. The nurse directs us into Dr Lyme's room. The dark-haired doctor stands as we enter. She has a serious, humourless face.

'Hello. Please sit down. How have things been since last time?'

Last time I was desperate. Last time I listed my struggles with the ointments, the day- and night-time bandaging, the vomiting, your refusal to drink. She studies the nurse's notes.

'This is remarkable. Louis has gained a significant amount of weight over a very short period of time.'

Her serious face is smiling.

I tell her that, yes, I have been following the foods she has instructed me to feed you. Turkey, vegetables and grains made into a puree. You continue to vomit most of it up. And then I add, 'There's another thing. I've taken Louis to see a Chinese doctor. He's given me herbs. They need boiling for four hours each day and they turn into a syrup and amazingly Louis drinks it up each time.'

She's on her feet, leaving the room. Her voice is furious.

'You can only back one horse.'

Dr Nook is more understanding.

'This is rather remarkable and I think as it's working you should continue for a while. I may even be able to postpone the operation if Louis's weight gain continues to improve. We'll do some tests on his kidneys. We need to check that no damage is occurring from this. It has been known for Chinese medicine to be filled with potent steroids.'

All your kidney tests come back fine and we continue to give you this medicine until your weight climbs back up onto the graph and the doctors' worries subside.

I should feel joy when Natasha is born and I do for a split moment but I'm soon filled with fear and dread of how I am going to cope.

It becomes obvious later that Greg and I will have to do things separately so that Natasha gets some time, some attention; the chance to be treated normally.

Right now as a baby she doesn't seem to notice our struggles. She has a happy personality, rarely crying. She is content to burble and play and watch as I care for you. She sits in her baby bouncer in a snug pink jumpsuit and wriggles her toes in her fleecy booties, she kicks her feet up and down and gurgles. Her blue eyes crease into half-moons as she watches you.

TWO

We take you to the Montessori nursery across the road from our flat.

'Would it be possible for Louis to come to the nursery and watch the other children play, just for a couple of hours a week?' *While I care for your baby sister. For us to have an hour or two's break.*

The nursery teacher agrees. 'Well, I'm willing to give it a try,' she says. 'I'm sure we could try an hour or two once or twice a week for you.'

They don't manage two hours.

'I'm sorry, we didn't realise the extent of his needs, his noise. We can't cope with him.'

We can only joke, 'Hey Louis, you've been expelled!' What else can we do? We are seriously worried. Who is there out there who can help us? *What are we going to do?*

⁓

The doorbell rings. It is Zoe, the physiotherapist from the hospital. You are sitting on my hip, your legs wrapped around me. I've picked you up from the floor. I've shoved your baby walker into the cupboard; she doesn't approve and I don't agree with her. You could either thrash on the floor unable to move or you could be in a walker moving around the flat.

'It will prevent him from gaining the will to walk.'

I went and checked with the orthopaedic surgeon at the hospital, who was straight with me: 'I've seen many children through the years when these walkers have been in or out of fashion. It has no bearing on the child's ultimate ability to walk.'

That was enough information for me but Zoe still doesn't agree.

You cling to me as she walks in with her confident gait.

'Ah now, let's have Louis.'

And I wish I could have known more at this time in our lives. If I had I would have shown her the door. She takes you from my arms and lies you on the Afghan rug on our living room floor, on your stomach and waves a toy above your head.

'Where's teddy, Louis?'

You are wriggling and starting to cry; now you start to scream.

'I think you are asking him to do something impossible.'

'No, it is important for him developmentally to learn to crawl.'

'But he can't even roll over yet.'

She perseveres and when I think about this now she might as well have been asking you to do a one-finger press-up.

When she left that day she forgot her file. I heard her footsteps descend the stone spiral staircase, the sound of the heavy storm door bang and shake. I'd scooped you up in my arms, your dummy in your mouth to comfort you, when

I noticed her file on the sofa. I don't usually look at other people's things but she's bugged me today the way she was with you. I open the folder. Her first entry is noted for that early clinic visit when you were only four months old, and two months if we take the doctor's corrected age. The one when she rolled you around on your chest while you cried.

She had written: 'Seen at outpatients clinic . . . mother has a tendency to over-baby infant.'

⁓

Some days your blond hair stands straight up around your gaunt oval face, your eyes wide spaced and blue. I manage to capture your alien look as you lie flat in the bath. You still do not have the strength to sit unsupported so I run the water not too deep. I lie you carefully down in the water so your head and body are covered, your face only partially so. The water frames your cheeks, your lips, your eyes. And your hair still stands on end. I crouch up onto the plastic bath's edge, place my feet on either side and point my camera straight down. And it catches you just how you are.

And the photograph will travel with us through the years as you grow and change. It leans against a wall in a frame and people who come into our lives are drawn to it, exclaim, 'I love this photograph. Wow, it's Louis? He looks like an alien.'

⁓

And here I am carrying you in my arms up to the clinic again. You are nearly three. I have not seen Dr Thompson since those early months after we left the hospital and here he is; we have met in the corridor again.

'Ah, Alison and wee Louis. How are you doing?'

He has a wide grin and a twinkle in his eye. I think he likes me as much as I like and respect him. I'm greeting him back, trying to smile, but I'm shattered. You are thrashing around in my arms, screaming as usual.

'That wee boy wants to be put down: he wants to run around,' Dr Thompson says amicably.

'Yes, but he can't. He can't stand, he can't even sit unaided.'

I see the shadow cross his face. The awkward end to our conversation as we both walk sadly away. We no longer need to wait and see. You have developmental delay in all areas.

In the clinic I ask, 'But what does this mean in the future? How will Louis be?'

'We still don't know: you will have to wait and see.'

'But you must know something, surely?'

'I'm sorry but it's very difficult to tell. You are being referred to the community paediatrician; the follow-up clinic at the hospital ends shortly. Dr MacAuley will start to put in place a number of professionals to come and see Louis to help him.'

⌒

I am in a cave in complete darkness. I am enveloped in
black, a black that does not touch but hovers around,
surrounds.

The despair and grief engulf us as we try to care for you, the constant pain and distress you are in. And your sister has come and I fear for her also. What have I brought her into?

'We should split up. You look after Natasha, then at least you can both have a life,' I say.

'That's not going to help, is it. We can barely cope with both of us caring for Louis.'

'But what is going to happen?'

Greg is silent

I am silent.

I picture the cliff. I picture jumping holding you tight in my arms, falling and falling through the air.

~

'Dr Nook – I've been researching various charities that can help children with cerebral palsy while they are young to try and reach their full potential. I've discovered one called BIBIC in Somerset that creates a personalised exercise programme for each child. It requires a referral. Have you heard of them?'

'Yes, I have, but there is a charity called Bobath with a centre based here in Glasgow. This is where our physiotherapists recommend a child like Louis to attend. I'm prepared to write a referral but it may take a while to secure funding and there's a very long waiting list.'

⌣

You are not improving. We have a list of doctors and specialists who inspect you and suggest things. Nobody is saying we have to wait any more, nobody is saying anything. Dr MacAuley has mentioned the words 'special school'. Your care is so intensive I can barely function.

THREE

My destiny has been decided. The realisation hits me full force in the stomach. I don't want this destiny. I don't want to be the mother of a disabled child. I don't want to be a carer forever; I don't want to lose my freedom. But I haven't a choice. My fate has been decided for me and it's a devastating feeling to know that this is it. No more wondering whether to do this or that.

Shall we emigrate? My uncle from New Zealand is visiting.

'That would never be possible for you now. They don't allow disabled children or adults into New Zealand. I'm sure it's the case in most countries, not unless you have the means to provide and care for yourself.'

And it's a good job you weren't born in America. Would you have survived? All the intensive care you required – we'd be bankrupt or you'd be dead.

And all my dreams, my possible careers; they've all melted away. I can't seem to do anything. I can barely get through the day; I am so fatigued with all your care needs. *Will this ever let up?* What I feel in my heart is so deep that at times it makes me gasp. I cannot accept this is happening but I've realised I have to. I've got to forget our early hopes and dreams; stop expecting you ever to catch up.

And it helps.

Now I think of the worst possible scenario and start from there. I imagine we will be stuck in this status quo forever, get no further than here. That you will never stop vomiting, never stop screaming, never sit unaided, never move around, never talk, never feed yourself, never dress yourself, never walk, never sleep through a night without waking at least five times and never communicate with me in any meaningful way. I expect nothing more than what we have. This will go on for ever and ever.

But you are making improvements, slowly, so slowly. And each little step that you make surprises my heart. It will happen unexpectedly, when I've long since given up that possibility for good: you will suddenly manage it.

Look, Louis! You are sitting unaided today.

⁓

And today another beam of light has pierced into my cave.

I rush into the living room to see why you're squealing. I'd only left you seconds before, propped up with pillows positioned around you keeping you safe and upright. I'd left you to go and fetch a toy from your bedroom to place on the wooden floor in front of you. As I dash back into the room I see that the pillows have fallen away and a space remains where you'd sat. You are shuffling across the floor.

You can move.

You are squealing in delight. Your legs are in front of you bent up at the knees and your arms are pushing down on the floor behind you and you're finally moving forwards. You stop and look up towards me. There is glee in your eyes and your mouth is wide open in an enormous smile.

'Wow, Louis, look at you,' I say in astonishment. And you squeal, turn and start moving again.

The effect of your bottom shuffling is miraculous. Something has happened inside your body because your vomiting subsides. Is it your stomach muscles? Do they strengthen from the movements you can now make? Instead of being sick you make long violent burps but the food stays down mostly and you begin to get stronger.

I've learnt something in life because of you: I've learnt what matters. It's very simple and it is something worth striving for every day. The fleeting feeling of happiness for whatever small reason makes life feel bearable. If you are unhappy it is impossible to be happy, so that is the key. Whatever keeps you content and stimulated, whatever enables you to communicate your needs, keeps you happy, and that makes me happy.

It's your pain and frustration that make life unbearable. The possible reasons are multiple and there are lots of things about you that I still don't know. What is the cause of your crying today? Are you hungry? Does your stomach hurt? Is your eczema itching? Are you struggling to breathe? Are you allergic? Which foods? Which animals? Are you feeling trapped, frustrated because you can't walk, get around, reach something? Do I not understand? You can't tell me, you can't speak, you can't say what you need. Later I'll discover you are desperately trying to let me know your obsessions, your terrors, later I'll discover acid burns in your stomach and causes you to vomit. Later I'll discover you have acute hearing, you are blessed with perfect pitch, certain sounds all around are overwhelmingly loud and they're piercing your ears as you cry.

But now in this moment of freedom you are happy, you bottom shuffle around the flat exploring in crannies. And in time you will get a rhythm to your movements, pushing your palms and your heels hard into the floor and bumping your bottom along the boards, you get quicker and quicker. You'll wear holes into most of your trouser bottoms even though I buy ones that are padded. When I pull them out of the clothes basket to hang them up to dry I will smile at the holes that need patching; you must lean to your left, as it is always the left buttock of your trousers that gets completely worn through.

FOUR

Today you start at Special School but you won't let me leave. I stay here for the two hours in the morning twice a week.

Your school is tucked behind a street of red sandstone tenements near the River Kelvin, surrounded by low stone walls with rusting metal railings. There is a high solid metal gate that opens wide to let the school buses in each morning. The large drive allows the specially adapted buses to draw up close to the main building's entrance. The back doors are opened and ramps clatter down to the floor. Escorts help push the children in their wheelchairs or buggies out to the smiling school staff who appear, wearing comfortable clothing. Friendly words of greeting ring out as the adults swap their care roles. The buses restart their engines and turn out of the drive and then it all goes eerily silent.

Around the edge of the redbrick building is mown grass with a number of blossoming cherry trees and a semi-complete raised garden area. As funds are raised, volunteers from the Duke of Edinburgh's Award scheme and the Army come in to offer their help to make the garden more pleasant for you children to use.

The building is one storey, old and dilapidated. There is a corridor that runs down its length with large airy Victorian classrooms positioned off it. At the far end of the building is a particularly large room. This is for nursery-aged children.

This is where I've brought you today. In time you will move up the corridor as you increase in age to enter different classrooms according to your disability. In between these two distinct areas is an office for the head teacher and a room for a doctor and a nurse. The extent of the disabilities the children have here requires daily medical supervision.

You arrive on your first day with your legs wrapped tight around my waist and my hands clasped together under your nappied bottom. You cling like a monkey and won't let me put you down, so eventually I sit down on the floor too.

In time the staff will provide you with a special chair and a standing frame with a tray. Both are on wheels and you are strapped in to play certain games, press buttons of animal sounds or put boxes on top of each other while trying to help your posture. You don't interact with the other children but you like to watch, humming on your dummy, squealing now and then.

One little girl befriends me. Each time I arrive she will sit by my side, stretch her legs out straight in front of her, wiggle her light blue shoes. She likes to smile up at me and offer me toys, show me her doll. Her name is Maisie. None of the staff discuss why each of the children is here at the school. With some it is obvious but with others it's not and I find that I wonder why they can't be at an ordinary nursery. Maisie is very able. She looks a little different: her head is slightly larger and her eyes are bulbous, but that isn't a reason to be here. In time I gather through observation of her deterioration and catching odd bits of conversation that

Maisie's condition is degenerative. She is here as a lively four year old able to speak, hear, walk and play, but within two years she will die, as one by one the things she can do disappear. The pain on Maisie's parents' faces is especially hard to witness. Every parent who comes here is in his or her own stage of distress. It makes it almost impossible to form any kind of friendship because no one wants to share or compare.

You sit in the nursery and cry and squirm and suck your dummy but as the weeks pass you begin to settle. Gradually you begin to bottom shuffle away short distances from me to watch what is going on elsewhere. You've been given a special assistant, Jean, to help you play and join in. Little by little I manage to move away, then sit on a chair by the wall, then sneak out of the door, until four months later you can be left. You still scream but it's manageable for them now.

I feel an enormous sense of relief the first day that I manage to leave you all morning in school. I walk out of the building knowing you will be fine. You will be toileted and fed and entertained for a few hours. I walk through the silent grounds, under the cherry trees and out onto the tarmac road. I wander right down to the River Kelvin and stand still on the bank, watch the brown-grey water flowing rapidly under the bridge.

I want to have another baby.

I know it seems crazy but I loved growing up with brothers and sisters. I feel lucky to have four siblings. Natasha has you for her brother, but she has no other sibling to talk with or play with, and no one to share her concerns with in the future about you and me.

I hope it can also bring further normality into our lives. Over time, Natasha has lessened the intensity of my pain. Her brightness has brought other children and adults into our lives and they've come to care about you too. Now I can listen to other mothers complaining about their children without wanting to cry, without my inner mind screaming that I'd give anything to be in their shoes. To have a 'normal' child has helped me, but what about her? And what about the new child I want to bring into this world? What if things go wrong again? If only it were possible to know that everything in any further pregnancy will go okay. When I became pregnant with Natasha we still had so much hope for your progress. I know there are no guarantees when having a child, but I don't think we could cope if something went wrong again.

Greg is worried. None of the doctors we have spoken to can explain why you are the way that you are, why you have not caught up after all, why you are not going to that normal school. Everyone has gone silent.

Greg doesn't want to risk it.

'I don't want to have another baby if there is any chance that there is some underlying genetic cause. The doctors don't seem to know why Louis is the way he is; what if it's something to do with us, our combination of genes?'

I speak with the paediatrician at your school, Dr Buchanan.

'Why is Louis the way he is? We want to try for another baby but we are worried in case this could happen again.'

'I don't know why.'

～

Audrey has died. She was your great-grandmother and a child prodigy on the piano in her day. I'm looking at a collection of newspaper cuttings after her funeral. They show announcements of concerts, photographs of her performing on stage, she was playing to royalty by the age of five, but she gave it all up when she married your great-grandfather Alan. It was front-page news in *The Times*, but no one remembers her now. It was Audrey's mother who made her play and I remember her telling me her mother had insured her hands. Audrey felt she'd missed out on a childhood so she had lots of children of her own to experience it again through their eyes. Now she has gone. I will no longer receive her spidery handwritten letters of encouragement that have been dropping through my letterbox about you. When I think of Audrey I see her face beaming from her bed, her wizened finger pointing to small oval gilt frames on her wall – a radiating circle of offspring, six children and twenty-four grandchildren and the circle was continuing;

the great-grandchildren were coming and you were up there on her wall with your shock of blond hair.

⌒

The annual Christmas family gathering is taking place at Len and Catherine's house. I've missed the last few since you've been born. We have travelled from Glasgow to York-shire and I am standing in the living room talking to my Aunt Janet. She is asking me questions about what happened at your delivery.

Janet looks across the living room floor at you sitting on the carpet. Your body is slumped forwards and your head is hanging down. Len is bent down beside you. I know he's checking you out for the first time. He'll come and speak to me later, tell me what he thinks as a paediatrician, though he'll soften his thoughts. Janet turns back to face me; her face is kindly but I can see concern there.

⌒

Dr Buchanan has referred us to a specialist genetic centre at Yorkhill hospital. We get an appointment in the New Year. Dr Gosse inspects you on the couch and watches you standing and trying to walk holding my hands.

'He's very thin and wasted. There are a few minor details that I've noted; nothing that appears to indicate anything obvious but you never know. If there is an obscure syndrome that I have not considered we may find out from this list of observations. I'll send away my findings and check the obvious ones too. In the meantime we'll take some blood and do further detailed chromosome checks. I'll be in touch when I get the results.'

'What are these congenital defects you mention?'

'Well, you say you were told by a doctor that Louis has thirteen pairs of ribs. This is very common. People all over the world are walking around with thirteen pairs rather than twelve and are totally unaware of it. But it is just one of the things that is different about Louis. And then there are the small teeth and his wide mouth. I note that Louis still has all his milk teeth and also he has a pigeon chest.'

'I've been told that is due to the pressure of the ventilator on Louis's soft bones when he was born. It wasn't there at first; it came during his time in hospital.'

'Yes, yes, you are most likely correct there, but it is worth mentioning all of these things just in case it brings up anything.'

We have thrown caution to the wind. The genetic tests are not back but I have got pregnant.

I'm terrified of anything going wrong again. I've been offered more detailed checks through this pregnancy and I can barely contain my fear at times. I arrive panic stricken at the hospital. The nurses know me, are kind and understanding. They check my blood pressure, they monitor the baby's heartbeat, and they give me a scan – I will be given so many scans this time – and then they reassure me and send me home.

~

Dr Gosse has called us back in to see her and she has another doctor with her, a paediatric neurologist called Dr Jalloh. I sit there pregnant while you bottom shuffle around her room. Dr Gosse tells us that there is nothing to suggest you have an underlying genetic condition; your chromosomes are completely normal. She's done detailed tests and everything has drawn a blank.

'This means there may be a one in four chance of it happening again.'

She must have seen my horrified face because she quickly added, 'This is what I tell any person when we cannot find any cause.'

It seems an alarming statistic to me.

'I've invited Dr Jalloh to come into this meeting as he might be able to help us in identifying the cause or causes of Louis's disabilities.'

Dr Jalloh invites us back to his clinic the following month.

'Can I take a detailed history from you about what you know about your pregnancy and Louis's delivery and his time spent in hospital?'

We discuss the bits that I know: the pre-eclampsia and placental abruption seen at delivery; that you were very light for your gestation and that Dr Thompson had told me you'd suffered no bleeds to your brain that he could see on the ultrasound scans.

'The only thing I can suggest that might help us further in finding out why Louis is the way he is would be to conduct an MRI scan. This will tell us if Louis's brain is normally formed, is of a normal size. It will also be able to indicate if any parts of the brain have been damaged.'

'When will this happen?'

'Ah, it is likely to take up to a year, there's a long waiting list and your son's scan isn't urgent, but hopefully it will give you some answers.'

And Greg and I nod at the doctor in the consultation room.

I still have unspoken hopes deep down inside that somehow, if we only try hard enough, you will miraculously metamorphose and recover.

⁓

It's been nearly two years since Dr Nook wrote his referral letter to Bobath. At last a thick A4 envelope drops through the letterbox with a long list of questions about your current abilities. At the end of the forms it asks me what we would like Bobath to focus on when they see you. I write down we'd like advice on exercises that may help you to ultimately walk. I post the forms back and two weeks later we are offered a six-week block of therapy to start in two months' time. My younger cousin, Sarah, comes up to live with us for a year, which is perfect timing. She will care for Natasha while I take you to the Bobath Centre for your sessions.

On paper Bobath appears to offer hope to any desperate parent with a child suffering from cerebral palsy. They offer intensive blocks of personalised therapy in the three main disciplines: physio, occupational, and speech and language therapy. I was so excited about taking you there; I couldn't wait to get some of their expert feedback.

But Bobath doesn't help you to improve. We attend two hours daily for six weeks. I was eager and willing to listen to any suggestions. You were bounced on a ball supported at the waist by one therapist while another lifted items into the air for you to stretch out for and another crouched down low, held your feet firmly as you scrunched up your toes and contorted your feet. They spoke in hushed serious tones to each other about your cerebral palsy in all four limbs, your lack of balance and your twisting feet. They noted your shrieking and felt you had sensory overload, observed the way that you continually bite your arm and wondered if you had a low arousal level and were doing this action to help stimulate yourself. *Yes, yes, and how can you help us?*

At the end of the six-week block they suggest some minor tasks to perform daily such as rubbing your feet with a bobbled cloth for you to experience texture and arousal. They explain that you need to gain an understanding of your place in space.

'And exercises: are there any regular exercises we can do?'

'It's the positioning that counts. There has to be correct positioning. We suggest that you hold Louis's feet flat to the floor while you distract him in play. When his foot curls you are to prevent it, hold it tight in the correct position.'

The feasibility of these suggestions is limited and the results from their initial six-week block non-existent. You are sent home with a typed report containing a series of correct positioning postures for your feet. Your helpers at school try their hardest to accommodate this for you. A learning assistant holds your feet in position for a period of time each day as you stand in your standing frame or sit in your special seat. It makes no difference.

Over time I've come to realise that their suggested treatments were well meaning but pointless. The 'correct positioning' theory ignores that cerebral palsy is a permanent disorder affecting muscle tone, reflexes and co-ordination. So some tendons are shorter than others, some muscles tighter or wasted. This causes pulling, contortion and deformity of limbs. Spasms and involuntary movements occur that cannot be controlled by will alone and no physical manipulation can alter positioning alone either. As you have grown, this fact has become more apparent. The pull in your shortened tendons has twisted your feet further. I discover in time that this happens. That cerebral palsy worsens during

117

growth spurts. That children with cerebral palsy can deteriorate and in their early teenage years, if not already, end up permanently in a wheelchair. I come to believe by your determination alone that exercise is the key. Forget perfect positioning.

During your second block of treatment at Bobath the three therapists agreed with each other that they didn't think there was any point in you coming for further treatment. They said there was no more that they could offer you. I was astounded, even though I still had so much to learn. *How could that possibly be?* You have so many verbal and physical needs; you can't talk, walk or even crawl.

But Bobath did help you in another way. One of the therapists noticed, as you babbled incoherently, that your noise was rhythmic, in time to the background music playing in the room.

'There's a charity called Nordoff Robbins. They offer music therapy to children with disabilities. Maybe Louis could benefit from them?'

~

The birch tree outside your window shimmers and a small group of starlings chatter on the branches. The sun shines through the leaves and into the bedroom casting patterns across the stained beige carpet, over our bodies. You sit legs bent backwards, resting on your nappied bottom. A pile of videos and their boxes are scattered all around you and you are shrieking, biting your arm, sitting back then leaning forwards pressing your face down onto the carpet, howling. I'm on my knees facing you.

'Louis, what is it, what do you want?'

Through the small opening in the large sash window fresh spring air touches my face, brushes it gently, crosses over my furrowed brows, reminds me of life continuing outside. Your scream becomes louder. I stretch out my arms, fists clenched.

'Is it the television? Do you want the television on? Yes or no?'

I shake my left fist for yes and my right for no. You lean forwards and, with a strength that you have mustered from deep within, hit my fists away.

⌒

A melodic Irish voice is trickling down the phone line; I can feel the vibrations of his voice in my ear that is warming with the softness of his lilt.

'Look, I'm telling you, I know I said I was full and had a long waiting list but I have to see him again. His response to music was incredible. We communicated together through sounds. I sense he's locked in and scared and I know I can help. I want to offer to see him in my lunch hour.'

*

119

The radio is playing Nat King Cole. His seductive voice is drifting around the kitchen, 'Quizás, Quizás, Quizás . . .' Natasha is in the highchair, plastic spoon in her hand, food smeared all over her face, and you are on the kitchen floor bottom shuffling around, squealing and babbling. I'm sure you're trying to sing along to the tune; your sounds have a rhythm to them. My belly is swollen again, not long to go. I'm leaning on a broomstick for support, feeling anxious, panicking about the future and feeling overwhelmed at all of your needs. I turn to Greg who is tapping along to the music on the kitchen table.

'Do you really think this is worth the effort? A one hour journey across the whole city for just twenty minutes, is it actually doing anything for him?'

You've been going for music therapy for a couple of months now after Brian offered to see you in his lunchtime. I haven't been able to take you myself; I can't carry your weight in my pregnant state.

'I'm not sure if it is,' Greg answers. 'Nothing much seems to happen. He just plays the piano and sings a bit and then says, "That's it, we mustn't hurry things."'

Screams erupt; you're prone on the floor on your back thrashing your body, banging your head hard, howling.

'Louis, what's wrong, why are you screaming? What is it? Hey, were you listening? Do you want to go, Louis?'

Your crying stops abruptly.

FIVE

Your brother Jack has been born; it's November and at last I feel that you can be you. I no longer crumple when I watch little boys play football in the park. I have one of those now. I know it seems wrong that it's taken this for me to be able not to wish you were different.

⁓

It is Natasha who reacts with shock when Jack is born. She gets down on her hands and knees and makes wailing sounds, crawls around the flat like a baby. You watch her incredulously then collapse with delight into giggles.

Natasha comes to find me when Jack is six days old. I'm in bed propped up on pillows quietly feeding the baby. Tasha tells me, 'You can give the baby back to the hospital now. I don't want it any more.' And this moment reminds me of you when Natasha was born. You came to the hospital carried high in Greg's arms. You did not want to look at the baby; you twisted your body away and squealed, lifted up your arm and pointed repeatedly, over and over, towards the hospital bedroom door.

⁓

Grace is in your class when you move up from the nursery to your first classroom. Grace's cerebral palsy is severe and she has to be tightly strapped into her special wheelchair and standing frame. She enjoys all the games in the class with your teacher Val and she is absolutely determined to try. Her body rotates and arms twist preventing her from doing the things that she wants to do, but she is managing to communicate her needs through pressing a pad on her tray and she clearly understands what is going on around her.

Dylan is also here. Dylan makes my heart lift with his cheeky smile. He's rather like you: he's thin and wasted, but he wears tiny steel-rimmed glasses and he's happy all of the time. He sits back on his folded legs on the floor and unlike you he can rise up on all fours and crawl. He likes to crawl over and speak to me if I come into class – unlike you and the others, he can talk. He smiles and cocks his head and likes to ask 'why?' to every answer in my reply.

Your teacher, Val, is a hoot. She has the widest mouth and smile and an enormous amount of energy to cope with all of the four children's needs in her class. She has an assistant, Trisha, and they like to call you 'Banana Man' because of your love of a mashed banana every day for your morning snack and your gesturing continually for more.

You've always loved bananas. I still can't quite believe the day last year when I barely dared to admit now how many bananas you ate. I had pushed you around the park as you squirmed and screamed and had sat in the grass under a tree with my best friend Rowan. I had a bunch of five bananas with me. While Natasha and Rowan's son Brody toddled around, you sat with your mouth held open wide and made a sound that meant 'more', as I mashed with a fork and then spooned the banana in. When I'd finished number five you'd continued to cry so I'd left you with Rowan to buy another bunch from a distant corner shop. When you reached number ten and still asked for more I had to refuse. And the strange thing was that your belly didn't swell. How that was I cannot tell.

⌒

We keep being told by the speech therapist at your school that your understanding is limited. She makes you use her PECS book, containing basic symbols of things that you need or want. There is a picture of a Weetabix, a cup and a banana for you to point to. No wonder you ignore her. No wonder you push the book away. You can make sounds for these things that I can recognise; you babble and I know what you mean. You refuse it at home; I can see that you want to communicate more.

You cannot read, well, not as far as I can tell. I read to you in your bedroom with picture storybooks. I try and help you to understand the words. I trace my finger along the pages in the hope that you will begin to pick up on what those words mean. And I've noticed you respond to rhythm and rhymes, particularly poems by A. A. Milne. I read you 'The King's

Breakfast' over and over, you love all the changes of voices, the king and the queen and the dairymaid and the cow; you are enraptured.

And your grandfather Spike plays 'video' with you when he comes to visit and help. He takes all of the videotapes off the shelves in your bedroom, takes them out of their boxes and scatters them across the floor. You love this game. You bottom shuffle around the room and match the tapes back to their boxes.

'What do you think?' Spike asks me. 'Do you think Louis can actually read?'

'I don't think so.'

'Neither do I, but look, he can link every tape to the right box so he can recognise through the letters and marks somehow which belongs to which. It's a start.'

Your arms wave in the air in spasms; your legs kick uncontrollably on the floor and your voice makes guttural singing sounds of excitement as you wait to play the game again. And now you like to be timed as you do it. Spike's clever like this. He can think up a game for you to play that is fun and exciting for you. How quickly can you match them all up? You squeal as you grasp each box and shove the tape in.

But you are cleverer than any of us realise. Look at what you have done with the school/home book. This book has become your form of communication with us.

It is a miraculous development. I didn't realise it at first.

Each night as I lie on your bed and try to read you a story you hit it away and shove your rolled-up schoolbook into my hand. You've rolled it up tight into a tube and I unfold and open it. First I read out what has been written that day for you in school and then I get out the pen to fill in what you have done that afternoon and evening at home. I read out the teacher's words and then I begin to write my own. You listen intently and make babbling noises as I talk.

'And then you did this, didn't you, Louis? You enjoyed playing a game of video with Spike and you put thirty tapes into their boxes in four minutes and fifty-two seconds. And then you had lots of mashed bananas and custard. I gave you three and you were pointing for more.'

After I've finished writing you pull the book off me and open it at the first page and motion that you want me to read it to you. You want me to read the whole book. As the book fills it takes longer and longer to read to you each night until I'm saying, 'Louis, Louis, I can't read the whole book, it will take all night. I'll read fourteen pages.'

And you take the book off me and pick, choose a page where you want me to start. *You see, we do communicate and we can communicate, you clearly understand what I say to you.* It takes me a while to realise that you are doing more than just listening to your daily life events recounted: you are learning the book off by heart. You need me to read it over and over again until one day you pull the book from me when I ask you what we should do tomorrow. You uncurl the book, turn over pages with your stiffened fingers and point to a page. I read it out loud and it mentions visiting Simon, Rowan, Brody and Ryan. You are getting excited, kicking your legs.

'Louis, do you want to go to Simon and Rowan's house?'

You tap my 'yes' hand.

⁓

And I find that I daren't open your bedroom door sometimes now in the mornings. I hover outside waiting to hear a hint of a noise from you. I find I am scared. You've not woken or called me at all. All is silent and quiet. *Are you alive? Have you made it through the night this time?*

⁓

You don't realise, you don't know that people are frightened or nervous or just a little bit unsure of what to say or do with you. They don't want to say or do the wrong thing and I can understand why. But you like everyone. You want them to see your book, the book that I write in every day and night. You want them to see it and read it out loud and they soon come to understand and then you want them to write something too. You want them to add their name and say something about themselves and what they are doing with you.

And people do.

I deliberately leave. I make an excuse. 'Just getting the cups of tea' or 'Just nipping to the loo.' It gives them time to be alone with you; time to see that there is nothing to be scared of. By the time I come back the relief is visible on their faces and the happiness on yours as they read out loud something shared and you giggle with joy.

That is what I have learnt: you have no capacity to judge. You do not notice other people's awkwardness; you just instantly like them, whoever they are, and if they will just help you communicate, you are grateful for their time. It's amazing how good that can make someone feel. Once upon a time a couple of friends – Cathy and Torston – were visiting and I lost them in the house. I found them in your bedroom sitting on either side of you. Both were beaming.

'We're just getting a bit of Louis therapy,' they laughed.

You have reached five and you still suck a dummy and I've started to feel a sense of shame that I let you, but what can I do? You appear to love them so.

I've started to pop the ones that I find around the house into the bin and let you see. I say out loud that maybe it's time to stop now, but your fingers wrap tight around the loop of the one in your mouth as I speak. You're not letting go yet. We are down to the last few in the house, then down to two and now there is one, just one always with you.

We are driving. You sit in your child seat in the back of the car. Your left hand holds the belt of your seatbelt tight.

You are sucking on your dummy making contented humming sounds. I look at you in the mirror and your face looks calm, your head is slightly turned to look out of the window. It is good to have you quiet. *Is that bad?* I begin to feel my body relax; I'm enjoying the peace of this moment. I hear the electric window lower behind me. I look in the mirror and your right hand is raised to your mouth, your fingers hooked around the loop and you pull, your lips suck and the dummy is out. You lift your hand to the window and let go.

'Louis, that was the last one.'

You don't register that I've spoken to you but make contented 'ahhing' sounds in the back.

⁓

For years I dream of you walking. You are standing upright walking towards me laughing and I am laughing too. I wake elated believing it to be true and within seconds realise it is not. Will you ever be able to balance? Will you ever walk? You seem to be too top heavy. Your legs are like sticks. *How can they possibly take the weight of your body above?* I think as the latest physiotherapist, Agatha, tells me again that you are not far off; it should come within months.

Your feet are small and very slender. They twist a little and your toes screw down tight when I try to stand you on the floor. You don't lift onto your toes like I've noticed other cerebral palsy children do, your feet stay flat but they roll slightly over onto their sides. The physiotherapists don't seem too concerned about this; they don't mention the visible difference in your feet to those of other children.

'He will be walking soon,' Agatha tells me again.

I so want to believe her, I so want her to be right, but I stare at your legs and your feet and I wonder how they will do it.

'You need to get him some proper shoes, though, to help him.'

I decide to push you into town and find a Clarks shoe shop. It promotes itself as the best shoe shop for children and today I want the best for you. We are going to do something mothers all over the country do when they take their children for their first 'proper' shoes. There is something that feels special and safe about Clarks, with its trained staff and its quality shoes, so I'm rather looking forward to getting you your first pair of sturdy leather shoes. I push your larger pushchair, used for children as they get older who still can't walk but who don't need extra positioning supports. This one will carry you for a couple of years longer before a wheelchair will become necessary. These are the realisation milestones we are experiencing from 'wait and see' to *this is what it is to be.*

The children's department is upstairs.

'Do you have a lift?'

'Sorry, no.'

'Can you help me?'

I walk backwards up the stairs as the assistant holds the front wheels. I push you over to the counter and pull off a paper ticket and wait for a shoe assistant to call our number.

'Number twenty-three. Hello, can I help you?'

'Yes please, I need some sturdy shoes for my son Louis, please.'

'Okay, we'll measure him for his size. Do you know his size?'

'No, I don't. It would be good to be measured.'

I've pulled off the soft shoes you are wearing and the assistant produces a foot-measuring ruler. She is crouched down and has positioned herself so that she can place your foot into it. She pushes your heel into the back of the mould and pulls the fixed measuring tape across your foot, slides the metal toe cap down to your toes. I see you curl them under your socks.

'Watch that,' I say. 'Louis is curling his toes; he does this.'

She talks non-stop telling me all about the importance of Clarks' training programme for its staff, the great importance of getting the shoe size absolutely right.

'I'll just go and find a selection for you. His feet are very slender so there may be a limited choice.'

You are making happy humming sounds. You are in a very good mood today.

The assistant returns with only one box and pulls out a pair of brown leather shoes. They look perfect. She puts them onto your feet and pulls the Velcro strap across.

'There. Now, please can you get your son to stand so I can check the positioning of his toes.'

I unstrap you from the pushchair and take your weight under your armpits, so you stand upright. Your body leans forwards and your legs are bent.

'Okay. Could your son just walk across the room now to check they feel okay when he's walking?'

'Oh, Louis can't walk.'

'Well, he has to walk in order for me to check that they fit him correctly.'

'I'm sorry, I don't think you understand: Louis can't walk.'

'Well, I'm sorry but it is company policy. We are not allowed to sell shoes without checking that the child can walk comfortably in them.'

This is insane. She's persisting.

I keep my voice calm and measured.

'Well, as you can see we have different circumstances. My son needs shoes to help him, but he cannot walk, not yet anyway.'

'Well then, why does he need shoes? Come back when he can walk.'

'What?'

That's it, I've lost it.

'Because he's five, for God's sake. What do you want me to do – push him round in his socks forever? It's cold outside – it's winter, have you noticed?'

'It's company policy.' She doesn't budge.

'I want to speak to your senior manager.'

'I am the senior here.'

We are back out on the street. I didn't handle that too well. I'm furious. Other customers with children had listened in silence. No one said a word. 'Fuck you all,' I'd shouted in my head. I carried you down those stairs by myself; my anger seemed to have given me strength. 'I'll be sending a letter of complaint to your head office and I'll never shop here again. You are talking a load of fucking shit.'

You giggled in the pushchair. You find it funny when people seem angry or upset. You seem to find the f word particularly funny; you appear to know it's a word I shouldn't use. You seem to know a lot given that you still can't speak. Is it my gestures? Are they comical to you? I often ask myself this when you double over in laughter at someone else's distress. I don't think it's because you are scared; you don't appear so. You seem to enjoy the drama.

How calm can I force myself to be? It just erupts sometimes. The stupidity! I try to remind myself that anger gets me nowhere, just eats away at me. It's just ignorance I'm facing. I could have handled that better.

But it's hard. It's hard sometimes.

⌒

Agatha refuses to sign the form that enables us to purchase a special walking frame with a seat, like a large baby walker. You are too tall now to use the baby ones, you topple out.

I've done my research; I've found a manufacturer with the exact product that we need. I was so pleased that one existed for you and I don't even want her to fund it. I just need her to sign the form as your physiotherapist to enable us not to have to pay VAT.

'I really feel that this piece of equipment is unnecessary, a waste of money. Louis will be walking within a few months. This could even hold him back.'

'But he can't walk right now. He cries most of the time; he's bored. This would help him to explore, otherwise he just bottom shuffles everywhere. Surely being upright would be better and may strengthen his legs?'

'Well, I'm not prepared to sign. He'll be walking within three months.'

I can look back now and tell you that didn't happen. You didn't walk for years and years after this. But Agatha never stayed to learn that she was mistaken. She was gone within the month. She'd moved on to a new post elsewhere.

⌒

The speech and language therapist is sitting upright in her chair facing us. She is talking in a high-pitched but soft voice. She has a well-meaning look on her face and her voice has a professional tone we are becoming accustomed to hearing.

'Your son has very limited understanding. It is understandable for parents to find this difficult to accept but we need to develop alternative ways of communicating for Louis. I'm afraid he is never going to be able to speak in the conventional sense.'

'But he's making babbling sounds, I'm sure they could become words. I feel he's frustrated at not being understood. It seems to be driving him crazy.'

'I suggest we continue with the PECS system, keep using simple pictures for Louis to communicate with us, basic nouns such as cup, shoe, teddy, which I stress he must be made to point at before you respond.'

'But I'm certain he understands more than this, more than we realise – we are waiting for him to have an MRI scan to tell us more about his brain function, but look, look at his schoolbook that I use with him, it's filled with detailed descriptions. He uses it to try to explain to me what he wants to do. And take poetry for example; Louis loves us to read him poetry at bedtime. He enjoys "The King's Breakfast", "Green Eggs and Ham". This picture system you use,' I hesitate, trying to find the right words, 'it's so limited, I think it frustrates Louis more than helps him.'

She looks at me in a pitying way. 'This is the way forward for him.'

A month later a letter with your hospital appointment arrives for your MRI scan. It's for mid-September just before you'll turn six. The scan will take fifty separate images of sections of your brain. I'm torn when the day eventually comes, Jack and Natasha are poorly with colds and I'm feeling under the weather so it's Greg who takes you. You have to be sedated I'm told later, you would never have kept still in that big booming machine.

SIX

I am carrying you down a green corridor of the type we've experienced in hospital, but this isn't a hospital. Your legs are wrapped around my waist and you're squealing, your excitement is bouncing off the walls and echoing down the length of the corridor all the way to Brian's door. As we approach the door flings wide open and Brian steps out. He fills the doorframe but it's his personality that envelops us. He is mid-thirties with a youthful face, gelled hair, a smart pressed shirt, pointed shoes and has a smile that is infectious. He greets us in his gentle brogue.

'Hello, Louis, come on in.'

You are doubled over in my arms giggling uncontrollably, shaking so hard you are unable to lift your head. I have never seen you happy like this. I wait for your excitement to subside, at least enough to be able to place you carefully down on a bucket-shaped plastic chair positioned beside an enormous drum. Brian sits himself down behind a large piano.

Brian begins to sing his opening song, a song that welcomes you while his fingers lightly flow across the keys producing a tune filled with crescendos. You have just managed to control your giggling and are sitting back in the seat with a wide smile that hunches up your shoulders and creases your face to reveal your tiny teeth. There are two drumsticks resting on the drum's skin and you lean forwards to pick one up. With one hand you try to hit the drum and Brian sings out to you as he plays to try two hands. You don't usually have the strength to do this. The drumsticks are heavy for you, your arms too weak, but you try and you manage to hold them both. You hold the drumsticks in both hands and hit the drum, not hard, just a light brush, and as you do Brian's voice sings louder. You lean back in the seat with your arms raised and your mouth open and emit a joyous cry. You try again and Brian's voice becomes louder still. I suddenly realise this is the only place you have ever had any control over the things around you. Brian begins to sing his song again.

'Hello, Louis, how are you today? Hello, Louis, how are you today?'

He continues to sing but when he comes to the word 'today' he removes it, pauses in the music, and then carries on. The room is filled with the sound of the piano and Brian's resonant voice and then a silence, and that is when I hear a whisper. Brian continues, pauses, and from the silence a word is formed from your mouth, floats out into the room, sweet, high and lilting.

'Tooo daay,' you sing.

～

There is a distant buzz of a lawnmower outside the frosted window. This Victorian brick building is surrounded by broken tarmac, concrete and tower blocks but there is one strip of grass that runs along the outside of the building. The hum is getting louder. I see you are distracted by the sound; it seems to have sent you into a trance. You have become stationary, your arms have dropped to your side and it is as if you have disappeared from the room. What has that sound reminded you of? Brian is playing and singing. He glances over and notices your sudden change in mood and although he continues to play he shifts the melody slightly, slows his pace and sings out a question.

'Are you happy or sad today, Louis?'

I have never asked you a question like that. You do not move, you make no sign to register you have heard except your body seems to expel air, sink down in the seat. You open your mouth and sing back a word. It whispers slowly from your mouth.

'Sad.'

I am in the kitchen and you are howling in your bedroom. I rush into your room to see what is upsetting you this time. Have you vomited again as you often do? You are sitting on the floor with music tapes scattered out of their boxes and the tape recorder in front of you. You are clutching your hands to your head and wailing. Your face is pink and tears are streaming down your cheeks. I'm down on the floor beside you.

'Louis, what is it? Calm down. You can tell me now, what's wrong?'

You're trying to speak, gasping for air.

'It's okay, breathe slowly, three deep breaths, that's it, that's better, much better.'

You press your hands hard against your head, look at the floor and speak hesitantly.

'Window. Birds ears hurt.'

⁓

I walk into the flat and place you down onto the floor. Greg pokes his head out of his music cupboard at the far end of the hall and then ducks his head back in. He doesn't speak and he doesn't offer to help. *What was that look on his face?* I shut the front door to keep you safe from the spiralling stairs – you'd shuffle out. I rush back down to get Jack from the double pushchair. I've had to leave him alone outside. Tasha is climbing the curving stairs slowly, little 'doggy' in one hand, the other holding onto the wrought iron struts of the banister. I'm back up to our flat and have left Jack sitting in the cot to keep him safe from you. I pass Tasha again as I head down for the shopping bags and the double pushchair. I need to store it behind the shared door. We are not going to be able to live here much longer. But everyone lives in tenement flats here so what on earth are we going to do?

I've just come from the local shops. We've seen Maureen in the Co-op – 'clappy clappy handies,' she always sings to you. Then we went into the 'banging shop' – we can't pass it without a visit. The first time we'd passed, you had pointed through the glass, made noises, wriggled your body. It was clear you had wanted to go in.

'Can I help you, my friend?' the shopkeeper had asked.

At the meat counter you'd doubled over in giggles, howling with delight while the man banged away chopping the sheep carcass into sections. He whacked his mallet against the enormous wooden block while you wept with laughter. We always buy our lamb from here now. I climb the stairs one last time with the bags.

Greg told me much later that he didn't know how he was going to tell me the news.

That evening when all the children are eventually asleep I come into the living room, sit down on the sofa. Greg speaks; he must have been waiting.

'There was a phone call earlier today.'

'Oh yes, who was it?'

I'm completely unaware what is coming.

'Dr Jalloh – he called about the scan. He said he'd studied the MRI imaging and wanted to explain.'

I sit up from my slumped position on the sofa. I'd have liked to have taken this call.

'What did he say?'

Greg looks away, his voice cracks.

'He's found damage.'

A letter will drop through our box a few days later explaining in clinical terms Dr Jalloh's findings. It will tell us that your brain is of a normal size with all parts present. It will tell us that this really rules out any possible genetic factor. In addition, it will tell us there is no evidence of bleeding, nor any evidence of chronic damage to the outer peripheral areas of the brain like the type that one may find in a child who has been born prematurely.

But then the letter will continue.

'Although Louis's brain is intact there is some detectable damage to Louis's brain in the high metabolising area. He's suffered a sudden period of reduced oxygen and blood supply. This has caused permanent damage to the Basal Ganglia region of his brain. When precisely, from the details I have here, I am unable to say.'

⌒

Your brain was perfectly formed, *perfectly*.

⌒

Brian is on the telephone.

'Alison, I hope you don't mind my asking but we think you would be perfect. There's a charity dinner and auction coming up for Nordoff Robbins. It's a big event, a great craic, and it helps to keep the charity afloat for the next year. Would you consider speaking at it for us? We like to ask a parent to share their experience of what the charity has meant to them and their child? You don't have to say much – just five minutes is enough.'

I hold my breath; I have a fear of public speaking. It is the bane of my life. I can't get up and talk in front of big groups of people. It's become a phobia. I blame it on the fainting incident when I passed out in the aisle as a bridesmaid at Catherine and Len's wedding years ago. Now I always think I'm going to faint when I stand up in front of others.

'I'd love to but I can't. I can't do public speaking, but maybe Greg will.'

'Sure,' Greg answers, 'I can do that.'

'Have you prepared your speech yet?' I ask Greg as the day nears.

'No, I don't need to. I'll just do it on the day; it's no problem. I'll just describe what Brian has done for Louis.'

'Don't you need to prepare something, though?'

'No, I'll be fine.'

I'd be useless and a nervous wreck. I love this about Greg, his confidence, his ability to perform, his ability to get up on stage and play his own music live.

We are sitting around a large table in a very grand room in the Glasgow Hilton. There is a stage, and a sparkling black backdrop surrounding us. Lights twinkle as if it were real stars in a sky. Greg leans towards me.

'Jeez, this is like the Oscars. I hadn't realised it was going to be quite so big.'

It's a black tie event and star studded. We've met Edwyn Collins in the lift coming down from our room. Wet Wet Wet have just performed, Deacon Blue are playing and Donovan is on later. I've not been out to a big social event in a very long time. My parents are up visiting to help. They've offered to look after all of you children overnight. We've been given a hotel room and it feels surreal being taken from the intense monotony of caring for you into the glamour of this night.

'Have you written anything down yet?'

Greg is looking a little bit worried.

'Bloody hell, I think I'd better try. I'm off up to our room.'

Greg borrows a pen off Brian and takes a napkin off the table and is gone.

This is an important night for the charity, a lot is at stake. I can sense the tension in the man beside me, the founder of the charity.

'You've managed to draw in many stars.'

He nods gently.

'How's Louis today?'

A short five-minute film has been made of you and Brian. A cameraman came and filmed one of your therapy sessions last month. They gave you a copy. You play it over and over at home, singing along to Brian. I think you like to see yourself on the telly, you like being a star. You still play it years later. It was shown on the television for Children in Need soon after this event and you like to share your moment of fame.

The compère is back on the stage and a white screen has dropped in front of the star spangled drapes.

'I think this is it,' I whisper.

The compère nods in our direction and Greg stands up. I squeeze his arm.

'Good luck.'

He walks up onto the stage.

I don't know how he can do this.

'And now we have come to the main part of the evening. What this is all about, folks. Please put your hands together and welcome Greg White, father to Louis – one of the children this charity has been helping. Greg is going to tell us all a little of what Nordoff Robbins has meant to him and his family.'

Applause rings out. Greg clears his throat.

'Good evening, everyone. I'll start by telling you a little about my son. Louis was born prematurely at thirty-two weeks, it was a traumatic delivery.'

Greg has paused. *Oh shit, he's sounding wobbly.*

'Unfortunately Louis was brain damaged.'

Greg is sobbing.

The compère whispers into his ear. The room has gone silent. I'm pinching my arm to stop myself from crying too. *Oh my god, Greg, you don't have to do it.* Faces turn towards

149

our table from around the room. The compère speaks.

'We are just going to play a brief film of Louis having his music therapy with Brian, one of our therapists.'

Greg has stepped back from the microphones and I can see the compère talking to him as the film begins to play.

The film is a tearjerker itself. Here you come. You are thin and frail and unable to balance, Greg is holding your hands. He is helping you to step-walk down that echoey corridor towards Brian's room. You are giggling with excitement – edit – there is Brian on his piano singing, welcoming you in – edit – there you are sitting on that plastic seat trying to hit the drum, turning the stick the wrong way up, putting it into your mouth – edit – Brian is drumming the piano with all of his fingers. A most beautiful high-pitched tune – edit – a look of amazement appears on your thin gaunt face as your and Brian's eyes meet.

Greg's returned to the microphones. He manages to talk. He tells us how you couldn't talk before we found Nordoff Robbins. How it has been a miracle for you and for us as parents to see our son unlocked by the power of music therapy.

The room erupts.

Greg walks back towards the table.

'I'm so sorry,' he says to the man beside me. In the background I can hear the compère beginning the auction.

'You've heard what we can do, the difference we can make to these children's lives. Now let's see what we can raise to help these children more.'

People are staring. Brian leans forwards to Greg. 'Don't

apologise, Greg. There wasn't a dry eye in the house. I predict a very successful night for us.'

'No, I blew it,' he whispers to me. 'I didn't realise. I've never spoken out loud about this before.'

In bed the next morning Greg is suffering: he's hung-over. I'd helped him stagger into the lift, collapse unconscious on the bed.

'What happened out at that bar then?'

'I had to get out of that room. When I got through the door there was a bar straight in front. A man in a kilt came through the door too. He drawled in an American accent that he wanted to buy me a drink. He told me my speech had moved him deeply. I asked him what he did. "Oh, I just write a few songs," he said.

'"Come on," I insisted, "you can tell me, what songs? I'm interested." I could see behind him a queue was forming, then I realised that queue was waiting to speak to me! "Oh just a few songs." "Like what?" I persisted. "Give me an example." "Oh you know, like that song, 'What's Love Got To Do With It?'."'

~

They're everything really, aren't they? All those things that we take for granted like being able to walk, play, write, get dressed, wipe our bums, brush our teeth, tie our shoelaces, chew our food, blow our nose, lick our lips. You still can't do any of these things. We help you to do everything and little by little, at a pace that is imperceptible, we make progress with some things. Others will never come. The damage is done.

⁓

I have to be brave for you and face the world out there. Face other parents and children. *It's okay, you can speak to us and we will welcome it. There is nothing to fear.* I try to be open and clear. I don't want Tasha and Jack to be unable to be invited to places too. I assure them it's fine; one of us can go and one can stay behind to care for you. Of course I understand that if you came it wouldn't work, because you just scream and cry and thrash and bite and I would be holding your hands, step-walking you around and around like a toddler although you are six now, or holding you, legs wrapped around me, as you repetitively pass me the folded-up five pound note that you want me to open so you can fold it up tightly again. If you came it would be a disaster.

⁓

I watch a documentary on Nelson Mandela. He's reading a newspaper on an aeroplane. He's folding the paper closed, lining up the sheets of paper meticulously, making the edges meet exactly, folding with extreme precision and care. The camera is stationary, watching. It takes him a very long time. Is this a coping strategy from his twenty-seven years of confinement? Has this meticulous precision arisen from

152

a need for some control? I see similarities in his behaviour with yours and your folded five pound note. Is it your years in and out of hospital, the pain you have suffered, being unable to speak, to move, to let your needs be known? Is this why you have obsessions and compulsions? Are they your coping mechanism with life?

We are moving. We can't stay in Glasgow any more. How can we? You are nearly seven and I have to carry you in my arms up stairs wherever we go. The hurdles are getting harder to manage the older you become.

Everyone lives in tenement flats in Glasgow and Natasha is about to start school. I can't see how I will ever be able to take her or collect her from there with you; there is a long line of steps right up to the main school door. And our landscape architectural business has plummeted. It's been impossible to run well with the amount of care that you need. We've been thinking hard about what we are going to do. How can we have a better life while all of you children are growing up?

So we've decided to move to the countryside. We've found a south-facing plot of land in a National Park in Wales. It's been for sale for ten years: we saw the sign long before you were born. As far as we can see it's the cheapest plot in the whole country. But the site has a lot of potential. There is an old stone cowshed and a largish grassy field. It's remote, but it is where my wider family have holidayed since I was small. There are beautiful beaches and surely there will be people to know, hopefully even some fellow artists hidden out there?

I hadn't thought we could consider going somewhere so distant, but Mary, your grandmother, has done some research. She has discovered that there is a special needs school in the nearest town and, not only that, it has 'Outstanding' for its latest OFSTED report. We will be able to live in my parents' tiny holiday bungalow while we build our home. We will build it to meet all of your needs. We will use our skills in architecture and design and try to give all three of you children the chance to be free. Tasha and Jack can run wild in the countryside while we care for you.

Well, that is our dream.

~

We have to get rid of the goldfish but there's no one who wants them. Yours is called Blue and Natasha's is called Pink, but we can't take them with us down to Wales. We've decided to slip them into the Botanical Gardens fishpond that we often go and visit. One of the glasshouses has a circular pool with a raised low stone wall and black railings fixed on top. Natasha and other small children like to step up on the wall and lean over the railings to look down into the water. They gaze down at pennies gleaming up from the bottom and watch goldfish and carp of all different sizes swim around through the weeds and the plants.

There's a guard who wanders the glasshouse and we wait until he has passed. You're sitting in your large pushchair and in its back holder we've got a plastic container filled with water holding Pink and Blue. I'm carrying Jack in a baby pouch strapped round my middle and I'm standing behind you holding onto your pushchair handles. Greg is trying to look oh so casual while Natasha is excitedly checking no one is watching.

'Okay, ready,' Greg says and I move out of the way and he grabs the container, scoops both fish into a net and plops them into the pond.

'There, done,' Greg says with relief.

You take no notice but we're all peering over the railings down into the water to see. Blue has headed nose down to disappear into the murky bottom but Pink (who is orange) has started to swim around the pool and Tasha is happily following her fish, walking around the wall. To all of our horrors a large carp suddenly starts to chase Pink. Natasha is screaming, frantically running around the pool, you howl. But as I turn I realise you are howling with laughter, collapsing into giggles.

SEVEN

We are in Spike and Mary's holiday bungalow in Wales. It is cramped and claustrophobic. Stuart, our actor friend, captured the chaos when he visited us from Scotland that first autumn. His black and white photographs show a scene of jumbled mess: piles of clothes, videos, books, Jack in a nappy, his toys scattered around him; Tasha dressed up with a feather boa around her neck dancing with Flora, Stuart's daughter; and you, bottom shuffling across the floor. Your favourite game right now is to pile all your video boxes up on top of each other and then to knock them all down. They are scattered all over the floor. Here you are again in the second shot, frozen mid-shuffle, but I can hear the noise, the squealing, the cry, the screams as you play your other favourite game – pulling Jack's hair.

There are only two bedrooms and you need one of them. Tasha or Jack can't join you; you thrash and squeal through the night. Instead we four are squashed into one double bed in the back room. Sometimes, in fact most times at the moment, Greg goes off into the back garden shed. It's not great for our relationship but what can we do? And now Greg is away. He's travelled back to Scotland to complete a design commission he'd started before we left. He is earning some money, keeping our heads above water.

Keeping our heads above water is not easy but we've been fortunate so far since you've been born, thanks to the ripple effects from our work before. I often wonder how on earth we could have got by without it.

Before you were born we had worked hard and saved our money to get onto the property ladder. We'd bought a flat that needed extensive renovation and as a result it became worth a bit more. We'd managed to save for the flat deposit through the landscape architectural business that Greg and I had set up. Back then we wished to design cutting edge urban outdoor spaces. In reality it was hard to get recognised for that kind of specialism, big firms got the work, but we were managing to get small commissions, gaining recognition, and earning enough to get by. We got lucky when we entered a design competition for a new town square in a distant small town in England and won. It was Greg who designed it, I had told him not to bother as it was so far away – I got that wrong.

The new town square was situated in front of a newly built Safeway supermarket, which had contributed towards the square's funding. At the official opening of the square we met the chief executive of Safeway who'd handed me his business card and told me they were looking for a landscape architectural firm up in Scotland. They were expanding.

I didn't call him. I didn't want to design car parks! But a week later the chief executive called me and offered to fly me down to London the very next day to attend a meeting to discuss contracts. I'd realised by then that this could actually be our big break, so I put my artistic dreams to one side.

We got work, quite a lot of work, and it became our bread and butter for a number of years. When you were born this work saved us. We were able to advertise and employ someone else to help us run the contracts. It didn't leave much money to spare but as our world came tumbling down, all around, as we were completely overwhelmed with your care needs, at least we could still pay our bills. The contracts kept dropping through the letterbox. Then one day a few years later, they stopped. A project development manager at Safeway had interfered. By the time Jack was born they'd practically all ended and then to finish things off completely Safeway was bought out by Morrisons – that was the end of our luck.

Our decision to move had been driven by this change of fortune along with our situation with your care needs. It was also at this time that Greg's mother tragically died very suddenly from her alcoholism. Greg inherited just enough money to buy the plot of land we were now building our new home on and we also bought the plot next to it. The plan was to use our design skills to build a home we could live in that would meet all of your needs and to build on the other plot to earn income through holiday lets. Our budget was very tight but then these plots were cheap so it was still possible. We hoped to design something special with these houses and it was a plan that could incorporate caring for you. Your needs and my exhaustion had made me unemployable – I would have had to take time off constantly and Greg felt he couldn't leave me alone to cope with it all, working long hours all the time. He needed to help, to stop us all falling apart.

⁓

There's a knock at the door, I open it and it's the plumber my parents like. He is a nervous man. I try to put him at ease but you can feel the ordeal he suffers when having any kind of conversation. He is thin and has short, thick black hair and large soulful eyes; they dart around as he fidgets, his voice is quiet. I know that he lives in a rambling house near this tiny village, alone with his mother. He doesn't talk much but he stares.

'Would you like a cup of tea?'

I leave him waiting nervously in the sitting room with you squealing on the floor and go into the kitchen to make it. As I carry the mug through the door on my return I find an unexpected sight. You have passed him every single video box you can find, stacked one after the other on his lap. The tower of boxes is swaying. I laugh but he doesn't. I help to lift them down. He jumps up leaving his tea and says he'll return when my parents are next down.

I tell the story to Greg a few days later when he is back from Scotland. You are sitting there on the floor; Greg is sitting reading the newspaper. I notice you pulling yourself up using the TV stand. You seem to be balancing yourself as I talk. Then I see you let go. You are stepping across the room.

'Daddy,' your high-pitched voice squeaks.

You step one, two, three.

'Daddy,' you say, louder.

You're going to make it; these are your first steps across the room to the sofa.

Greg lowers his paper and looks.

'Daddy, fucking hell!' you say.

⁓

Your sister Natasha has a happy disposition. She is always smiling and creatively busy, dressing up and dancing around, a ray of sunshine, as she chatters and talks. Today is her first day at school in the nearby village. I stand and watch her at the school gates. She walks up to two small girls; they are the only girls in her class but they turn away and ignore her and she troops a few feet behind them. I can't bear to watch. There are five children in her year group including herself; each classroom consists of three years yet this still only comes to fifteen children in total. They sit at three different tables according to age and the teacher gives work to each group. I hope Natasha may pick up more information from these classes if she overhears the older children's work.

A few weeks later I get a telephone call. It's Natasha's teacher – she wonders if I can come in to discuss Tasha's progress. *Will they tell me she's gifted?* At the school the teacher tells me they are concerned: Natasha is developmentally behind. *What?* My beautiful intelligent daughter, your sister, is not as able as her peers, it transpires. When they hear she is still in nappies at night I see concern flash across the teacher's face. 'It's impossible to deal with this right now,' I try to explain. I leave with them arranging for a nurse to speak with me in a few weeks' time. I go home reeling. I have failed her.

'We are going to have to take this nappy off,' I tell Tasha and I get plastic sheeting and a single mattress. I make her up a small bed on the floor. It doesn't take long to succeed and I feel shame at my lack of parenting.

Later Tasha does well at her schoolwork and her singing voice is a rare gift. People will ask, incredulous at our kitchen table, 'Is that Natasha?' as they hear her exquisite voice drift through her bedroom floor in our new house.

EIGHT

Kevan, the builder, is reluctant to let us move into the new house. It's taken eighteen months of gradual work but we are there: it's the week before Christmas and it's ready. We've had to be careful, the budget was tight; but we've enjoyed it too, sourcing things, hunting things out. We've had to oversee everything as it all came together but it's done now. It's in a good enough state to move in.

'This has become like a baby to me,' Kevan tells us. He's been passionate about the build. He lives three doors up and he's been building the house in the evenings and over the weekends after his day job has finished.

'It's the first house I've ever built fully,' he has told us numerous times. And he's been perfect; he's meticulous and obsessive and does everything well. When Len visited in the summer he'd studied the frame and had been taken aback at the jointing in place. 'This is pure craftsmanship,' he'd said in astonishment.

'We need to move in, Kevan,' I gently tell him. 'It's ready now.'

It is dark when I wander up to find him and break the news. I've found Kevan inside lying prone on the floor. I can see through the glazing that he's lying down. He's holding a torch in his hand and has rolled onto his side. He's shining a light over the wooden flooring. He jumps and sits up as I pull on the door handle and slide the door open.

'Ah hello, Alison. I'm just checking the floor's all level, that there's no lifted boards.'

The floor is immaculate. The light ash wood is shining; it's been carefully varnished a number of times.

'Kevan, it's looking amazing and it's also hardwearing. It's going to need to be with us coming in – you know what we're like as a family!'

Kevan nods sadly.

'Yes, I was thinking, maybe I should add another coat of varnish? Are you sure you want to move in before Christmas? It will be a bit of an upheaval for you.'

'Yes, we do. We are going insane in the bungalow. We need some more space.'

'I'm going to miss this house.'

'I know. You've put everything into this for us and we are really grateful. You know you will always be welcome to pop in anytime, don't you?'

Kevan hangs his head.

We move in the very next evening. The door is rolled back so that we can step out onto the timber deck of the garden. You are standing in the main open plan space: the heart of the house. It's a sunroom, a hall and a living space all in one. You are standing in your walking frame squealing as the boxes are being carried in. Kevan appears.

'Hi, Kevan, the big day's arrived at last, heh?' I'm smiling.

'Yes,' he says. 'I've come to see how you're getting on.'

'Thanks. Come on in. We're just getting all the boxes into the hall and then we'll start to unpack.'

But I notice he's not listening to me – he's staring at you, his face ashen. You are banging your walking frame up and down, up and down, on the perfect ash floor, like you do.

~

'Do you think he realises?'

'No, he doesn't seem to.'

'No, I don't think so either.'

I am discussing toilet training with Mrs McBride from your school. You seem to make no connection with your pushing and grunting and filling your nappy. We try to get you to the toilet in time but usually we are too late. You are eight years old now.

'The only thing we can do is remove the actual nappy,' the teacher advises. 'He needs to feel the discomfort. Hopefully after a few accidents at school and at home he will begin to register and we'll be able to get him out of them at least in the daytime.'

And so we have had a whole school year of toilet training. I send you into school with two pairs of spare trousers and pants and the soiled ones come home in a plastic bag. I have the washing machine on constantly. It used to be for your bottom shuffling: your trousers are covered in holes on the backside. Now at least you use your walking frame most of the time. At least you aren't shuffling in your poo, although you do in the morning. I have to leap out of bed the moment I hear your waking noises. I know you are going to slip down off your bed, start shuffling over the floor. You can't walk with your frame once your shoes are off, so you bump down onto the floor and you're off. I know you like to empty your bowels first thing in the morning around six.

'Louis, wait for Mum,' I call as I race down the stairs, hear your happy whooping sounds, then the sound of a thud down.

Damn, I've missed you again.

I'm going to have to clean up the mess and it's so much harder to get you clean now you've bottom shuffled over the floor. It's leaked out of your nappy, into your pyjama bottoms, smeared down the inside of your legs. But you don't seem to care that it's spread everywhere. I've found you putting it into your mouth before and so has Greg. That time Greg couldn't hold the pain in, had broken down and sobbed in front of you. Later you will ask him, 'Why did you cry then, Daddy?'

I put the bath on again.

⌒

We've travelled all the way from south Wales to Liverpool to determine the type of cerebral palsy you suffer from and the journey has been hellish. We have booked a hotel for the night. The room is far too hot. You have been agitated the whole journey and have just violently vomited onto the carpet. Now you are silent. I use the internal telephone and call up the hotel staff to ask for cleaning materials and a bowl. There is a knock at the door; a young slender man in a uniform enters with a cloth and some air freshener, no water. He scoops up the sick with one cloth and then rubs the remains vigorously into the carpet with another.

The next morning we arrive at our destination. We abandon the wheelchair at the bottom of a narrow flight of stairs in this Georgian terraced house of hired offices. You are eight years old but still slight to hold. I carry you up in my arms; vomit weakened, you cling to me, nappy heavy under your trousers, legs wrapped around my waist. We pass an ashen couple at the top of the steps, a child in their arms too, its cerebral palsy obvious to see. We knock and a voice says to come in. As we enter I take a few steps but you are wriggling hard so I bend to place you onto the floor and you are off, bottom shuffling towards the doctor, squealing piercing sounds of greeting.

Half an hour later we walk down the busy street pushing you in your chair. You are whooping and your legs and arms are flaying up and down. Rumbling buses and cars pass close by and their fumes spread over us, but it is just noise and smells to me of the life we are no longer a part of. I have my head tilted up to feel the warmth of the sunshine on my skin.

'I don't understand you,' Greg says. 'This is hard to digest so why are you smiling?'

I tilt my head sideways, look at Greg and smile again.

We have to take these moments.

'I'm enjoying feeling the sun.'

NINE

We are taking a train to London. You have been studying the London underground map for so long that I've decided it is time that we go. I want you to go on an underground train. You are nine years old and I can still just about lift you. I can push you in the extra-large pushchair and lift you out when I have to. If I don't do it now we will never be able to again. You will wrap your scrawny legs around my body and I will hitch you up onto my waist, although you are getting rather long. My sister Rosie is going to meet us. We will go on the trains together. I will carry you down the escalator and stairs and she will fold and bring down the pushchair. Together we will manage to give you a day in London.

We've caught a train to Paddington Station. I've got your nappies and a nappy bag. You are rather big to balance on the toddler-changing mat in the train toilet but that is what I have to do. I've got thermos flasks of mashed warmed food for your lunch and tea and yogurts for snacks. I have an overnight bag for you and for me because you are going to spend the night with Rosie and I am going to visit my friends Marc and Ishbel for one night. I'm going to have an adult evening with old friends while Rosie has kindly said she will look after you.

I have no idea if we will manage the day. We got on the train at 7.23 a.m. and will arrive at noon. You are clutching your A–Z of London with a Tube map on the back; you have been excitedly saying all the train stations you'd like to visit.

'We could go to the Natural History Museum too, Louis. How about that?'

'No,' you reply.

You don't want to see daylight.

At Paddington Rosie is waiting. She helps me with my bags and we leave them in the left luggage, head towards the underground station. At the top of the stairs we meet our first hurdle: I'm going to have to lift you down to the underground entrance. At the entrance I find a station guard and he radios for assistance. While we wait we chat and he hears how you've come all the way from Pembrokeshire for this special trip. You pass him your rolled-up A–Z and kick your legs up and down with excitement. This man has a kind air; he is the stereotypical station guard in a children's book, round and jolly.

'I can see you are going to have fun,' he says. 'Let's help it happen.'

For the rest of the day we are met at platforms, helped up stairs and escalators. On each section of our trip a station employee appears to be waiting for us.

'Where are you going to next?' they ask and then radio through to the next stop to warn them we are coming.

As I leave you later at Rosie's flat I ask her, 'Are you really sure you will be all right tonight?'

Rosie grins. 'I'll be okay for one night,' she says.

'Well, you have my phone, I'm not far away, just call me if

176

not.' And I disappear into the night.

When I arrive the next morning Rosie looks tired.

'Well, I didn't get any sleep!' She's still grinning. She comes back with us to Paddington, helps to carry our bags. We get a taxi, though; neither of us has the energy for underground trains any more. As we walk towards the platform I feel a hand on my shoulder. I stop and turn to see the kind guard who helped us yesterday at the start. He is holding a cardboard tube in his hand.

'I've been watching out for you three,' he says with a big grin. 'Here, Louis, this is for you.'

When we get home we unroll it – it is an enormous Tube map, the real thing. It is even dusted in soot.

⌒

I can't remember the exact day that your soiling stopped but it did. The clothes came back in your bag unused. It had taken nine months, a full school year, but we got there in the end. Now we just have the night-time nappies to get you out of. I think that can wait a while, though. I need a break.

⌒

You love repetitive phrases. Is it the musical ring that certain words have or something comforting in knowing I will respond? I don't know, but there are certain groups of words you love me to say over and over again and I hear you saying them softly to yourself in your bedroom like a song.

'I'm tired now,' you always call out to me.

'Have a long sleep now,' I have to say back.

I cannot answer in any other way. I cannot miss out one of the words or change the phrase or your anxiety will rise, panic entering your voice as you repeat your phrase over and over demanding the proper response. This is all harmless and easy to live with. The irony isn't lost on me, though; you fight being tired and will resist sleep at all costs. You will never allow it ever to be suggested that you are actually tired. As your head nods and your eyes flutter closed, if you hear those words, 'Look, he's tired,' your body will jolt upright and you will scream, 'No I'm not!'

It's no problem at all for me to reply to your favourite phrase in this way, but it is a little confusing for others and impossible to explain quickly the game that you play. Whenever you see me first thing in the morning or when I come to collect you from school or just at any impromptu moment, you will turn your face up to mine and say in your lilting voice, 'I'm tired now.'

And people will hear.

'Ah, is Louis tired?' 'Are you tired, sweetheart?' 'He's tired, Mum.'

'No, no, I'm not tired!' you scream back into their faces, hard. And then you repeat the phrase to me pleadingly and I quickly reply, 'Have a long sleep now,' and you go totally quiet.

Today I roll out a long sheet of paper on the living room floor. Natasha wants to do some colouring in and I've suggested that if I draw around her body on the paper she can fill it all in, make a girl the same size as she is. You watch and when I've finished drawing around Natasha you get down onto the floor and bottom shuffle over and squeal and lie down too and I draw around you and then Jack comes into the room and lies on the floor and I draw around him, so now we have three large sheets of paper with body outlines that can be scribbled on. Natasha colours hers neatly and Jack scribbles on his and you hold a pen and attempt to scribble on yours. Natasha looks over and sees that you need help so she moves over to your body shape and gives you a smiling face and some ears.

⌣

Greg has taken Jack fishing and I have taken you into town with Natasha to go to her favourite shop, a toyshop that, among other things, sells quality small plastic animals. Natasha has been buying the horses for a while now from this wide selection and each Saturday I allow her to choose three or so more for her collection at home. In the shop you watch and wait as she chooses. You don't want anything yourself but you enjoy going up to the till afterwards and paying the money for her, folding the note up tight.

All of Natasha's horses have names and she agonises over which ones to choose in the shop. When we get home she disappears upstairs to play happily for hours with them up on the landing. She lines the horses up all in a row and moves them around in circles, creates a stable and fields and puts small people onto their backs to ride them. She's safe upstairs on the landing away from you but you decide to bottom shuffle up the stairs to see her. She can hear your bumps as you move up the wooden stairs and she starts to scream for me to come quickly.

'Go away, Louis,' she says to you as you giggle; she knows if you get any closer you will knock them all over.

TEN

Today is your birthday. You are ten and you are squealing with excitement as I push the large wrapped box across the floor towards you. You manage to rip off the wrapping paper and look towards us to help you with the cardboard. It is a Henry Hoover. That is what you wanted.

You sit on the sofa and watch me vacuum around the house preparing for your party, your arms flailing, your legs beating up and down with excitement. We say your parties are the best because so many adults come to wish you a happy birthday. Family and friends from all over arrive with their children who run loose in our house and garden with Natasha and Jack. You sit on the sofa with the adults, ignoring them. Today at the party Greg picks up his guitar and starts to sing. Dave, the 'Clint Eastwood looking' builder, saunters out to his car and returns with his own guitar to join in. They sing a catchy made-up tune about hoovers. You shriek with delight at the words they sing alternately to you.

'Excuse me.'

'Do you have a hoover?'

'Where do you keep it?'

'Under the stairs.'

They sing over and over and you begin to join in, we all do, as it builds in harmony, peaks to a crescendo. You collapse over in giggles, barely able to breathe, but whenever they try to end the song you cry out, 'Again, again.'

You have been receiving an interesting collection of photographs recently. They have come through the post from family and friends posing with their hoovers. We have even received a photograph from our diving friend, Kate, of her hoovering up the seabed for her research. This is your latest obsession, your latest question whenever you meet anyone new. You hold out your hand and grab theirs and you don't let go. Your speech is still difficult to grasp but it's getting clearer.

'Hello, I'm Louis.'

'Hello, Louis, nice to meet you.'

'Do you have a hoover?'

'Sorry?'

'He wants to know if you have a vacuum cleaner.'

'Oh, right, yes I do.'

'What make is it?'

'It's a Henry Hoover.'

Right answer. You double over with laughter.

And you've started to work out where most people keep them, I discover, as I'm wheeling you through the local DIY shop.

'I need the toilet.'

'Do you really, Louis?'

'Toilet,' you say, louder.

The uniformed shop assistant who just passed us has stopped and retraced his steps.

'Excuse me, did I hear your son just say that he needs the toilet? There aren't any in here but I could take you to the staff one if you'd like?'

You smile at the young man. I bend over your wheelchair whispering.

'Louis, do you really?'

'Yes!' you scream clutching your crotch. 'Do you have a hoover?'

'Sorry?'

'Do you have a hoover?'

'He likes to know what make of vacuum cleaner you own,' I say.

'Ah yes, I do. It's a Dyson.' The young man is leading the way as I wheel you through double doors into the back section of the shop where it becomes more cramped.

'It's just a bit further on your left,' he says. 'I'll wait here for you.'

As we reach the toilet door your arm shoots out. Your hand, like a claw, clamps to the doorframe, forcing me to stop.

'Hoover.'

'Louis.'

'A hoover.'

You are looking transfixed at an upright vacuum cleaner stored in a corner right by the toilet door. You don't need the toilet at all.

185

I am driving Jack and Natasha to school. We are leaving the village and winding down the long narrow road that burrows between raised hedgerows dividing ploughed fields; a stream on the right-hand side winds with us. I look in the car mirror and can see Natasha and Jack in their school uniforms. Between them sits Edie, Liz's daughter, a pretty dark-haired girl from the village who is between their ages. Edie and Tashi are talking about names for horses and which is their favourite horse at the local stables.

'I'm going to have to go away later today, only for a night. I'll be back tomorrow,' I say.

'Why?' Jack wails.

'I need to go to Scotland.'

'Why? I don't want you to go.'

'I have to go to Scotland for Louis. You know how Louis needs help with things? I have to go to a meeting about how he will be cared for.'

I hesitate. Natasha, Edie and Jack are quiet in the back. I look at them through the mirror.

'And Tashi and Jack, I want you both to know that you don't need to worry about Louis when you both grow up and leave home. Dad and I will make sure that Louis is cared for and looked after when we are dead and gone. You two can go anywhere you want in your lives when you are older.'

It sounds a little American but I mean every word. This is what I want. Of course Tasha and Jack will love you and will worry for you and care for you, but I don't want them to be held back from having a life of their own. I don't want them to feel the weight, to be responsible for your daily care needs.

'Mummy, when you're dead I'll shoot myself,' Jack's voice rings out from the back.

I look in the mirror, startled.

Natasha looks over at Jack who has the biggest of grins stretched across his freckled face.

'Why, Jack?'

I'm totally bewildered.

'Then I can come and see you.'

Tasha rolls her eyes. 'Ahhh, Jaack, you're so stupid.'

Jack's not listening to her. He's grinning, looking into the mirror at my eyes; at this moment in time he means every word.

And how do Jack and Natasha understand and deal with your disability? I have always tried to explain your behaviour to them so they understand you can't help it. You can't help it when you double over with laughter when they fall and hurt themselves. They used to look shocked.

'It's not funny, Louis,' they'd shout, indignantly.

But they understand now that you don't mean it unkindly. You don't seem to understand other people's pain; you find their howling hilariously funny. Natasha and Jack now treat you like a younger little brother even though you're the oldest. They are kind towards you and help you. But most of the time they get on with their playing as you show little interest in joining in.

One day Jack comes home from school angry. A boy called Robert had been mean about you; he teased Jack about having a disabled brother. I had tried to prepare for this, had explained to Jack and Natasha that this might happen to them and to tell me if it did. I went down to the school straight away and talked with the headmaster and asked him to tackle it in a positive manner somehow. I don't know exactly how the headmaster handled it but he did it well because that is the only incident in Natasha and Jack's playground lives when you are used as a tool of aggression against them. Interestingly, years later, they have never forgotten the incident or the mean boy's name.

As you all grow older I'll notice that Natasha and Jack choose friends who are inquisitive and interested in you and your habits, the kind of children who want to come up to you and say 'hello' and ask you questions. I don't know if Natasha and Jack have chosen these friendships carefully but I'm pleased. Natasha's best friend is called Megan and Jack's is called Jamie. Jamie's got a mischievous sense of humour and appreciates yours. One day in the future Jamie's father Mike will tell me rather proudly what Jamie has said to him.

'He said, "Dad, if I ever get rich, I'm going to buy Louis an escalator for Christmas, because that's what he tells me he wants every year."'

We call it the wall of fame. Blu-tacked onto the wall opposite your bed are photographs in cardboard frames of everyone kind enough to take you on Megafobia at Oakwood, the local theme park. Most of the photographs show the person screaming and you laughing or else looking rather serene. It makes me smile every time I see it. My favourite photograph is of my younger sister Jenny. Her dark hair is blown back, her red lipsticked mouth is open and her magnificent cleavage is fully displayed as you both plunge down the highest drop on the ride. And I wonder now, how did you discover that place? I can't remember, but it's become somewhere that you long to be taken to. If anyone visits it's the first request you make, as my heart sinks.

Greg's managed to wriggle out of going. He has suffered from epilepsy in the past so he can't go on rides, which means that I draw the short straw in coming too. I need to muster all of my energy to take you, as it is physically exhausting. The thought of the hills I will need to push you up through the park, the toileting and the difficulties in feeding you, the queues and your overriding excitement and determination to stay until the park closes. But we are fortunate: the management at the park have made a rule for the disabled. This rule will be taken away in the future but for now it still exists. You are able to go on any ride twice without getting off. This helps enormously with the physical effort of lifting you in and out of a carriage.

Today we are heading straight for Megafobia. I've done your toilet stop and we've taken the tiny train into the site. I have lifted the wheelchair out of the carriage, helped you to balance out of it too and into the wheelchair. Your cousins Daniel and Adam are charging off towards the Pirate's Ship; Tasha and Jack are following them but Ollie is frightened and John's trying to cajole him, while Sarah is holding Lucy's hand as she pulls in the opposite direction towards the Umbrella ride. We agree that it is going to be impossible to stick together.

I push you along the tarmac path and hold on tightly to the handles of the wheelchair as we go down the steep hill and then stretch out my arms and back to push doubly hard back up the other side. I can hear the sound of Megafobia's carriage wheels on the metal rungs fixed to the groaning wooden frame. I can hear the screams, the rattle as the carriages turn a bend, the sound of a rush of air as they drop from a great height down and up again. You are whooping with glee.

We are allowed to enter through the exit route. This route is ramped up to the exit platform at the end of the ride. I push you up the steep ramps as the ride is in action. This helps to get up to the top before the horde of thrill-seekers are rushing off the ride to run around the paths to join the queue again. We stand to the side behind a barrier off the platform and wait. The carriages arrive back with a sudden braking halt as the riders laugh and shake their heads.

A man running the controls steps out from his small cubicle and calls across to us from the other platform.

'Not on this one or the next, I'm afraid.'

There are people queuing on his side of the platform. They are spaced along the platform in pews ready to enter the carriages once they have emptied.

'Where would you like to sit? I'll reserve the space in two go's time.'

'Where do you want to sit, Louis?'

'The front,' you mutter into your lap.

'Sorry?' the man asks. 'Where?'

'Louis would like to sit at the front.'

'Okay, mate. I'll save that one for you.'

The man jumps over the platform to help me balance you into the carriage. We both take your weight and lift you into the seat. I sit beside you and the bar is lowered.

Oh shit, do I have to go through this? I used to love rides but not any more, I've lost my nerve. I scream most of the way round while you are silent, holding the bar with a far-away look on your face.

'Phew,' I say when we get to the end. 'Are you wanting that second go?'

'Yes,' you reply.

'Do you need me to stay on with you?' I'm feeling sick.

There's a pause.

'No.'

'Are you sure?'

Pause.

'Yes.'

'Okay.' *I suppose you seem safe behind that bar.* I get out, my legs shaking.

'Same again?' says the man.

Your arm is outstretched. You want to shake the man's hand. He offers it to you and I know that your grip will be tight.

'What's your name?'

'Mike.' The man is smiling down at you.

'Are you on Facebook?'

'Yes, I am.'

'Will you be my friend?'

'Yes, sure I will, Louis.'

And you release him.

You are back from the second go.

'Okay, all out. I'll help you lift Louis.'

Mike is bending down, lifting the bar, placing his hand under your armpit and I'm standing over you on the other side. You make no attempt to shift your weight for us.

'Come on, Lou,' I say.

'Again.'

'Again?'

'Again.'

'Okay,' Mike says. 'Just one more time.'

Mike nods at me. Your words shoot out quick and clear.

'Five more.'

'You what! Five, mate? You're a chancer. Two more.' He's laughing.

'Ten.'

Mike's shaking his head. He's looking at you and up at me. I'm shaking my head at him, *No!* Mike has a strong handsome face, tattoos up his arms, a muscled physique. He straightens his body, leans back and looks at you with a grin.

'Man, you are a card. You can stay on all day.'

Oh no, don't say that!

And so you do.

I stand on the platform, and then I sit in your wheelchair as I wait.

'Is it safe? Will it kill him? How many rides can a body take?'

'Ah, don't worry about it. There's the rollercoaster society, they come every year and they try to set a new record. I was here once when they did over fifty rides.'

'Fifty!'

I lost count of how many times you went round but it was well over thirty. In the end Mike had to pretend to shut the ride in order to get you off.

⌒

I get a phone call from Jack's school; they want me to come in. This feels like déjà vu except the teacher and primary school are different. The new school is down the coastline with more children per class. We've moved both Tasha and Jack to this school to be able to make some friends. When I arrive the teacher gives me a leaflet entitled 'Gifted Children'.

'Jack is exceptional at maths,' she says.

I'd already guessed that.

Jack's been disappearing across the road to see Dave, the builder. He's only just six, but he carefully climbs the scaffold and talks to Dave as he breeze blocks the walls to a new house opposite. Jack watches Dave with his cigarette stuck in his mouth and talks to him about numbers. How many of those does Dave smoke a day? A week? And then he calculates how many that means a year. How old was Dave when he started smoking and how old is he now? Dave appears at our house with Jack in tow.

'Jack's bright, isn't he?'

'Sure is,' I say.

'He asked me about my smoking. I felt bad about him watching. I told him each cigarette knocks ten seconds off your life. I only meant it as a deterrent but he's calculated my demise. He said I should be dead by now.'

⁓

The large man leans out over the counter of his van and stretches his thick hand down to yours. You pass him your tightly rolled-up five pound note. You are paying for our chips. We came down to the far side of the village when we heard the boy racer horn. We see some of the old locals have come out from behind their net curtains and formed a queue. We'd heard the rumour too: 'There's a new fish and chip van coming to the village on Friday evenings. The chips are good.' When it comes to our turn to pay you grasp at the man's fingers.

'Hello, I'm Louis.'

'Hi Louis, I'm Martin,' Martin's voice shouts over the hum of the engine and the sound of the spitting fat.

You grin and squeal the tune 'La Cucaracha'.

'Do you like my horn, Louis?'

'Yes.'

'Do you want to press the button for me?'

You are overcome with giggles. I balance you with your frame over to the front door of the van and Martin lets you in. You press down and hold. The horn blasts out over and over. It hurts my ears.

'That's enough now, Louis,' Martin shouts.

I have to tug your hand off the button.

'Can I do it again?'

'Yes, sure you can, Louis. Come next Friday and you can play it again.'

And now you are hooked. When you hear Martin's horn in the village you want to go straight to the van. You shriek in anticipation, your excitement mounting through the week the same as my dread. I like and appreciate Martin's kindness but it's not how I want to spend my Friday evenings. I feel mean, you enjoy it so much.

Spike has been walking round the garden with you looking for spiky plants and stinging nettles; this thrills and scares you at the same time. You want to touch them but you know if you do it will hurt you; it is a game that the two of you like to play. Spike's thought again of something original that will entertain you, keep you occupied for a while. You are using your walking frame and slowly following him around the edges of the lawn.

'Look, Louis, here's a thistle,' I hear Spike say. 'Do you want to touch it?'

'No,' you scream.

I have snuck up on the two of you from behind the barn living room wall. I want to capture an image of grandfather and grandson. The look on your face when you are with Spike is one of intense concentration, thought and delight, but I don't want either of you to notice. I capture the image – a look of scared rapture, the likeness in your faces as you both look intently at a thistle.

I often joke that you are your grandfather Spike re-incarnated, although Spike isn't dead! You seem to share the same interests and he's so patient and caring with you. He has always been one of those crazy types. He runs over mountains and he cycles long distances. I'll never forget the evening he arrived to see us a year ago. He'd cycled all the way from Sheffield on his bike in a day. That's over 300 miles. He set off at one in the morning and arrived at the house at nine at night.

'How did you do that, Spike?'

I have visions of a bullet hurtling in the dark over the moors and mountains down through the valleys. He just grinned.

'Well, I ran out of steam near the end. A bridge was closed and I had to do a 15 mile detour but the rest was okay.' Spike's bike is leaning against the wall outside and he has a cup of tea in his hand in the kitchen; he's still wearing his cycling gear.

'When I set off I climbed up to the top of the tor then went over the dark peak. I stopped at the top to take a break at about two in the morning. It was a lovely still night. I met some young people up there. They were having some kind of a party. There was loud music playing.'

'Yes, Dad, that sounds like a rave.'

They must have thought they were hallucinating.

ELEVEN

We are going to try to find a bike for you and then you will be even more like your grandfather. We are going to drive all the way to London to try some out. I've been researching. There's a compound in a park on the south side of London where you can try different disabled bikes.

Oliver is talking gently to you as you sit in your wheelchair in the park compound. He's been showing us all of the types of bike that you could possibly ride, helping us to work out which would be best for you. The bikes take a while to adjust in length and height before you can try them and we've been standing here for over an hour while Oliver tries to get the latest bike right.

'This is an adapted recumbent bike and I think this might be the right one,' Oliver says, lifting his head up briefly.

We've already tried a double bike where we sit side by side but only I pedal, and another that was rather like a bucket truck with you sitting in the front. Both were heavy, cumbersome and disappointing.

'It depends if Louis will be able to pedal on his own,' Oliver is saying. 'I think that he might, and it can also be attached to your own pedal bike and pulled so both options are there. This bike was designed in Germany. They really know what they are doing there.'

You continue to watch as Oliver uses his spanner and

tools and we lift you in and out to assess, then move and adjust. At last he is ready. We lift you in and twist your feet into the stirrups. I try to wedge your feet into the metal plates but they keep twisting out, it's impossible. In the end we half-strap them in with Velcro and decide there's enough there for you to be able to push, and we put on your seatbelt straps. Oliver has tied a rope to the back in case you take off. It is going to require you to use both your legs and your arms at the same time and to look out for people. That's a concern: you don't really think about others, do you? In your walker I have to hold on tight to the back if we go into a public place or you'll just mow down anyone in your way.

You've started to shake. Your voice bleats out, 'I'm scared.' You say it again like a cry, 'I'm scared.'

'You've got nothing to be scared of, Louis.' This is Oliver.

You look up at him and seem to hear him but then you say it again while your legs start to shake up and down, up and down.

'Look, Louis, the worst thing that could happen has happened to you. There's nothing to be scared of.'

Ouch, that was frank. You don't understand him. You don't register what he has just said.

'I'm scared,' you just say again.

'I'll push you,' Oliver is saying. 'As I push, your feet will move round and you'll come to see how to move your legs. And I'll call out to you how to move your arms.'

He is patient. Your face is still as if in shock as you register the new sensation: the movement in your legs as your feet move round on the pedals. Your hands let go of the steering handles at your side. They are held out in surprise as you move down the path. Oliver leans over you. As he pushes the bike from behind he steers with the handles too; your legs move slowly around and around as he talks soothingly, reassuringly. Half an hour later Oliver says gently, 'You try steering now, Louis,' and he takes you away again.

'I think I'll fix it up onto a normal bike, then you can pedal and pull Louis around the park. His legs will go round and in time he will learn.'

It's a winter's day and Greg and Jack have gone down to the beach in warm puffy coats. When they arrive back at the house Jack runs into the hall and his face is radiant.

'Dad's going to make a sculpture with me.'

Greg follows Jack in and is carrying a bag filled with round plastic bottle tops and under his arm is a plank of driftwood. They spend the afternoon sticking bottle tops onto the flat plank and now it hangs on our wall in the central area and we can look at it from the kitchen table. There are many circles stuck onto the wood in all sorts of colours: red, blue, orange, green, pink and yellow and in all different sizes.

Later that evening when you're all asleep and I'm sitting down in the living room with Greg he tells me about a special moment down on the beach.

'The sun made it warm in that sheltered spot behind

the big rocks. We scrambled around on the pebbles under the cliff finding bottle tops. There was this moment when Jack stopped still and his little face looked up at me. "Am I dreaming, Dad?" he asked me. I answered, "No, Jack, this is really happening."'

It is Christmas morning and today for the first time ever we will go out as a family of five together on a fun activity. I treasure the photograph of that day as we all ride around the block, Tasha on her bike, little Jack on his, and Greg pulling your bike attached to his. You let out high screams of excitement and joy. You start to sing 'la la-ing' sounds as we go. Here we all are, together, doing something that ordinary families do. You can see in our faces: we look elated.

Ade the Blocker laid blocks for the house that was built next to ours. He would turn up in a bright blue Jag and get out with a wide grin on his face. He had a twinkle in his eye and a natural swagger and there was not an inch of fat on his sunbrowned torso as he laid the blocks. He was a brilliant storyteller, he had a colourful history to put it mildly and Greg enjoyed his company but I would keep my distance.

Ade has told you that he lives near Oakwood and has a view of Megafobia from his living room window. Ever since you've heard this fact you've been pestering Greg to take you over to visit. It's a year since the building work finished and Greg's suddenly agreed. Ade has rung him up with a design question about his garden so Greg's going over to look at it for him and said he'll take you too.

When you both get home later Greg raises his eyebrows, blows air out of his mouth and shakes his head at me. I stop wiping the table and wait in anticipation – for what? I'm not sure but I know something's happened.

'Louis enjoyed himself. But that poor kid.'

'You've enjoyed yourself, Louis?' I ask.

You whoop happily.

I've enjoyed myself too, I think quietly, the peacefulness in the house even though it's been busy. I helped Tashi and Jack construct a stall on our driveway; we used an old broken door to create a makeshift table and covered it with a tablecloth, placed cupcakes baked yesterday on the table's top and then drew up a colourful 'Cakes for Sale' sign and stuck it to a piece of board down on the roadside. Then I've tidied up the house and sorted out washing, and been cooking a bolognese for our tea in the kitchen. The house has been ringing in silence. All I've heard is small waves of chatter and laughter drifting up from the driveway. Now I'm standing still and curious, with a hand on my hip. I'm looking across at Greg and down at you in the hallway, waiting to hear what you have been up to.

'Ade asked me out into his garden; he needed me to look at a bit at the bottom. It was too awkward for Louis so I left him in the living room with Ade's teenage son Mark. I told him to call me if he had a problem. When we came in they were gone. Then I heard Louis. He was in their bathroom asking Mark to wipe his bum.'

'Louis! You know you must ask us for those kinds of things.'

You know but you take no notice of me. You're bottom shuffling across the floor to your bedroom humming a joyous tune.

⌒

I wake and it's gone. Usually I wake with a stab in my heart. You are eleven years old and the pain has disappeared. It didn't fade slowly; it has just gone. I've woken and I feel nothing but a lifting feeling in my heart, optimism for today.

The realisation that I have at last accepted what has happened feels like a lifting of weight from my body, my mind. It carries me above all of the tasks and the chores. I really don't care any more what anyone else thinks. I hadn't realised that I had but I must have. I don't care if an old school friend shares the fact that I am the one to have the disabled child. I didn't want you to be demeaned. I didn't want you to be described in that way. I didn't want you to be whispered about, discussed as something tragic and sad. I did not want to be seen as a victim. I did not want people to feel sorry for me; I didn't want any of this. I know people can't understand, how can they? I wouldn't have been able to and it's impossible to describe. I've just had to be stoical and now I genuinely do not care. What is this feeling? It can only be acceptance.

Greg is not there yet. I can still feel his trauma, see it etched in his face.

⁓

'You don't seem to want to go ahead with the operation?'

'It's not that. I just want to be absolutely sure I understand the procedure. How it is necessary and may help Louis.'

This is my third meeting with Mr Rhys, an orthopaedic surgeon. I'm sitting in a chair in a bare, strip-lit office. Mr Rhys's chair swivels as he leans onto his desk. He is a large man smartly dressed in black and has a kind warm face. He's studied you three separate times now on a hospital couch and always reached the same conclusion: there's a risk that you might lose the ability to walk in time. Your feet are getting worse, are twisted right over onto their sides and your stepping has already deteriorated.

I've asked if it is possible for a nurse to entertain you for a short while so that I can actually speak with the surgeon and hear his answers.

I ask my questions all over again and he's reassured me that this really is the best option for you. Mr Rhys has explained that there is a real risk that if we don't do the operation your ankles may fuse. That the contractions and contortions that you suffer from may become permanently fixed affecting your flexibility, causing your walking to worsen, your legs to bow even further and force you into a wheelchair permanently.

'The thinking is that by moving the tendons from one side to the other it will reduce the strength of the pull and lead him to be able to place his foot flat onto the floor. This should enable him to walk better. He may even in time be able to lose his walking frame. He will always be unsteady but he may be able to walk unaided or with poles.'

Is that really such a possibility for you?

I have decided.

'Okay. I'd like us to proceed with the surgery.'

Mr Rhys has even suggested that we attempt both feet at the same time to limit the stress of the operation and time spent in hospital.

'I'd rather do one foot at a time just in case things go wrong.' As I say the word 'wrong' my body shivers. *Please, please don't let anything go wrong.*

'Splendid. We'll do the left leg first as it's the most badly affected. You'll get a letter through the post with a date for the operation.'

TWELVE

Philip in the local Dr Barnardo's shop calls you his most discerning customer. The shop is on a steep hill that makes it slightly hard to get into, but I try. I push you up the hill in the wheelchair, my arms outstretched and legs pushing hard, then I have to get you up and over the awkward step and into the shop.

Philip comes out from the private back section.

'Hello, young man, how are we today and what can we get for you this time?'

You grin so hard you can't speak for ages so Philip keeps talking.

'Now let me see, sir. Is it steam trains you are looking for? You mentioned them to me before? Now I'm just popping into the back as I'm sure I put something aside for you there.'

He comes back. 'How about this, sir, a book on steam trains?'

'No,' you say without looking.

'Ah, that's a shame.'

Philip wanders around the shop pulling out items and displaying them to you in your chair.

'No, no, no,' you say each time.

Eventually Philip stops, puts his hands on his hips. 'Well, sir, that really is all that we have for today. I'm afraid we'll have to continue to look out for things that you want. Is there anything you would like me to add in my special book?'

'Yes,' you say with an enormous grin.

'I'm ready, sir, what shall I add?'

'A dredger.'

'A dredger?'

'A dredger and a steamroller.'

'Yes, sir.'

'And an escalator and a double bass.'

'They're all written in. None of these items come in very often, sir, but you never can tell. I'm sorry there is nothing for you today, sir.'

'Steam train.'

'I'm sorry, sir? Did you say you want the steam train book today?'

'Yes.' You're giggling.

You always want the very first thing, but you pretend, make Philip go through the whole shop first.

'I must say, a very good choice, sir.'

You've been given a room this second time. Eight days ago you had your first operation. Then we were in the ward. You'd been in a bed and I'd lain on the floor with an inflatable mat. On day five after the operation Mr Rhys had opened your cast and looked down at your foot, pausing.

'I want to operate on Louis again. The tendon is still pulling his foot over, I need to move more.'

You'd gone back in to surgery again two days later. And
now it hurts. You cried through the night for the last two
nights so they've moved us in here on our own. Now we are
waiting to be told when you can go home.

You lie in the bed and I sit exhausted by your side in a
chair. There's a telly up high on the wall and CBeebies is
playing. You watch the Tweenies on the screen lapsing in
and out of concentration. The room is hot. I try to open the
window to breathe some air from outside. The food trolley
comes by. I've explained about your food allergies and in-
ability to chew, so you get mash and beans and a yogurt. It's
placed on a tray on a table pulled over your lap. I help to
spoon-feed it in. The pain relief has been increased and it
seems to be working: you are only whimpering.

Your foot is raised up into the air in a plaster cast and I
can see your small toes poking out at the end. The hospital
physio comes in to see you. She is friendly and bright faced
like they've all been so far.

'Now it's important to keep Louis's foot raised if you can
for the next six weeks. Then when the cast is taken off you
will be able to begin to exercise him. Get him back up onto
his feet.'

We are sent home three days later. It's a relief stepping
out of the hospital into fresh air, wheeling you down to the
car, lifting you into your seat.

We make a contraption to keep your foot raised. The

hospital wasn't allowed to provide anything to take home with us and the local hospital physiotherapist has told us that she can't provide anything either.

We are hopeful.

Six weeks later we return to Swansea. You scream in fear at the sound of the plaster cutter. We need to cajole you, distract you and eventually hold you still while your cast is sliced down the side and removed. Your white shrivelled leg appears and we are told we can go home now, that you should get back to normal shortly.

'Are there any physio instructions you can give us?'

'No, just do what you usually do. He should make a full recovery.'

I'm a little surprised. I try to get hold of the paediatric physiotherapist at our local hospital to discuss what we should do but it is the week before Christmas. She's away. She will not be available until mid-January.

You develop a urinary infection that Christmas. We need to lift you to do anything. You are afraid and unable to bear your weight. You are barely sleeping and neither am I.

I call the hospital but there is no one available. I curse that it's Christmas, New Year. Eventually I get through and demand to see Mr Rhys at his next clinic in January. He's not very forthcoming.

'It will come in time for Louis, you just need to be patient.'

'But I understand that it's important to do exercise early

for a better recovery. Surely you must have some exercises that could be suggested?'

'No. This is not our remit here. That should happen in your own local area.'

Toileting has become a problem. You are permanently in the wheelchair and unable to get yourself onto the toilet. I have to partially lift you while encouraging you to stand on your good leg. Thank goodness they didn't do both at the same time or we'd really be stuck. *What was the surgeon thinking when he suggested that?* My back is killing me from all the lifting and I'm finding it incredibly difficult to clean you properly.

Today Faith, the children's occupational therapist from the local council, has come to visit us at home. I requested a referral over two months ago and I have been asking on the telephone ever since for someone to visit.

Faith stands in our hall looking stylish in an embroidered blue linen dress, her blond ringlets resting lightly on her shoulders, her face serenely blank. It is the first time we have met. I'm exhausted. You had me up six times last night. My sense of relief that at last someone has come is evaporating. Her face is immobile. She doesn't seem to understand what I've just said to her, that your risk of infection is even greater due to your hypospadias, that it's important that you are kept clean.

'He'll soon recover. It's not necessary to get you any sanitary cleaning equipment. Anyway, you'd have to apply for a grant because of the expense of a Clos-o-Mat toilet so I would not be prepared to recommend it. By the time it comes through he won't need one.'

'What do you mean? How am I supposed to clean Louis?'

'He can learn to do more himself.'

'I'm sorry? Before this operation Louis couldn't wipe himself and that was when he could partially balance.'

'You need to allow him to try.'

She's statuesque in her gaze. It's unsettling. I'm starting to seethe.

'Let me show you.'

We move from the hall into the bathroom. I wheel you through too. I keep you fully clothed but lift and manoeuvre you on and off the toilet seat, get you to stand precariously on one leg to demonstrate how I'm trying to wipe you. You are as helpful as you can be, but it's back-breakingly hard work. You sit back down on top of the toilet seat with your arms and legs flaying unpredictably around as your throat releases spontaneous cries.

'Do you see? It's not possible to clean Louis properly.'

'It requires you to stop doing it.'

She's gone too far, the heat is rising in my face. Faith's face is as smooth as a white stone gleaming on a pebbled beach. Her body is still and she keeps her gaze calmly fixed on my contorting face. I don't see a flicker of emotion in her eyes. I straighten up from my bent stance and I try to keep my voice calm but I can hear it is shaking. Her insinuation that the fault is mine has thrown me; in my anger I'm furiously trying to hold back tears that are threatening to erupt.

'So tell me, how do *you* expect him to wipe himself? He can't stand. He has cerebral palsy in his hands. It's not going to go away.'

Greg's heard my raised voice and has appeared behind Faith by the bathroom door, looking puzzled.

'Oh, he can do it if you train him. He needs to be made.'

'You're not making sense. We've been trying for years. He can't do it.'

She turns away.

'What about now? We need help.'

'I may order an additional bar for holding onto. I'll see what I think when I get back to the office.'

Greg's as incredulous as I am. He's turned pink. As she moves past him he growls, 'I'll write to the newspapers.'

She ignores him.

'We will complain about this,' I say as she goes out of the door.

Until now I've never wished our experience on anyone. I never thought that I ever would, but at this precise moment I wish it on her. I wish her the whole whammy, all of this, for it to swallow her, swallow her up whole.

I write a letter of complaint to her department but I'm met with silence. Eventually I get an answer to my phone calls. I am told Faith is on extended leave. 'She's in New Zealand,' the secretary wistfully says, 'and there's no one to replace her to deal with her workload right now.'

Much later, in the distant future, I'll regret my exhaustion that prevented me from pursuing my complaint further. Who else has she demoralised at their most vulnerable? But right now I'm desperately tired. I have to concentrate my energy; I need to find a solution to our problem urgently.

And I do.

What we need, it transpires, is a Bio Bidet. I can't believe it when I find such a brilliant thing exists: a self-cleaning unit built into a toilet seat that costs a sixth of the price of the Clos-o-Mat toilet and it does exactly the same job. The salesman tells me these Bio Bidets are all the rage in Japan and the Middle East but that here in the West we prefer paper.

It looks like any other toilet seat but is thicker and has a hidden retractable nozzle and a remote control unit to operate it. A nozzle extends and squirts or sprinkles water for as long as you wish, then it can blow you dry afterwards too.

You suffer a urinary tract infection while waiting for this equipment I've ordered and I try one more call to the occupational therapy department. I am told you have been removed from their list. If we want a new assessment to be made we will have to go through the process of gaining a referral from the hospital paediatrician again. I know the doctor is on sick leave. Anyway, it is clear – what is the point?

I give up.

I sit down at our kitchen table and stare out of the big glass window and see the trees lining the end of our garden bending from strong gusts of wind. I look at them bending and righting and realise that unlike them at this moment my trunk has split. We were just about coping before but this disastrous operation has sent us over the edge.

You are waking seven times in the night screaming for me. What can I do? If I ignore you it might be a time that you need your inhaler. I can't risk it. When I come downstairs and ask you, 'What is it, Louis, what do you want? It's the middle of the night,' you say you can hear humming in the walls.

I'm begging the doctors for help but I just get blank faces. They have separated you out with your learning disabilities from a child who suffers mental issues. They just can't deal with you.

You cry in pain. You ache in your joints, in your hip and your legs, and it's all because you are immobile. And Mr Rhys is unavailable. I'm told he can't see us again until April or maybe June. I'm making repeated requests for urgent physiotherapy but I'm told that this needs to be instructed by the surgeon. I ask Mr Rhys's secretary to please ask him to write requesting help for us but he doesn't. Eventually the local physiotherapist Jan Williams gets back from an extended holiday and examines Louis. She makes her opinion clear.

'Louis does not have a problem physically. He should be able to walk again with his walker.'

'But he can't,' I explain. 'He's in pain and he can't stand up straight.'

Jan provides your school with large leg splints that are attached to both of your upper legs for support. She's instructed your school support assistant and other members of staff on the importance of you exercising down the corridor. She suggests to them that it is insisted upon; that when you come to leave the building each afternoon to get onto your school bus you must walk. She instructs the staff to ignore you if you fall down or complain. That it is all attention-seeking behaviour that needs to be discouraged. She hasn't told me about these instructions; she clearly thinks I'm part of the cause.

I get a phone call from a neighbour.

'I don't know if I should be telling you this or not but I felt worried just now when I walked past Louis's school. Louis was outside, on the ground crying. He'd clearly fallen from his walker but the staff were ignoring him, talking over him as he tried to pull himself up.'

I'm blazing. My anger bursts through my exhaustion when I call up the school.

'I demand a meeting and an explanation. Louis is to remain in his wheelchair at all times in school until this has been sorted out.'

I am sitting in a chair in an airless meeting room at your

school. A round table is taking up most of the space; the chairs are filled with efficient faces, some are smiling tightly but their eyes are empty. They are nodding to each other, shaking their heads, writing things down. I am being offered pills: melatonin, Vallergan. I am being told your problems are psychologically induced.

'There really is no reason why he should not be walking in his frame again by now.'

'He needs to be forced, ignored if he falls to the ground.'

'This often happens when they reach this age, losing the ability to walk. You need will and perseverance; often it's the parents who haven't got it.'

'There is no reason why he cannot weight-bear; you don't need any additional toileting and bathing equipment.'

'You really must sedate him, his anxieties need to be managed.'

The tears are silently running down my cheeks.

'Look! Look at mother.'

Heads swivel and stare.

'She needs an assessment.'

They are all nodding.

⁓

Greg goes to the next meeting.

'You'll have a one parent family on your hands if you don't do anything. Two hours of help a month is pathetic. We're at breaking point. I'm going to leave, then you'll have to do something. You're going to have a child in care before you know it.'

He hasn't told me what he has said. He tells me later with an angry laugh when I tell him what had happened today. A social worker has arrived at our house to see me.

'I just want to make an assessment of how you are managing.'

I repeat to her how our sleep is broken constantly through the night; tell her about your pains, our despair at trying to cope.

'Do you get suicidal?'

Oh my god, this is humiliating. What business is that of hers? Do I have to say yes to get help?

'I'm not in a position to be able to offer you any respite, that's another department. But I will be suggesting to the children's services that you do need more than two hours a month. They should be sending someone out to assess Louis again shortly but I'm here to assess you.'

Tears are streaming down my face again. It keeps happening; I think it's the exhaustion.

'There is a possibility I can find funds for you to attend couple counselling if you feel that would help?'

'Sorry? The problems are with caring for Louis not between ourselves.'

She looks at me strangely. I consider her suggestion.

'Maybe we could do with some individual counselling to discuss how we are coping?'

And how do we share this agony? My heart howls silently, Greg's bursts out like fire.

And we argue, we argue about the noise, the distress, what the hell this is doing to us all.

And the darkness deepens.

⌒

I dream that one day we will have the help that we need today; that one day we will be saved from this struggle, exhaustion and despair. One day we can die peacefully because we will know that you will be provided and cared for, for the rest of your life.

⌒

You stopped holding your folded five pound note and moved on to a notebook. You would go over to people and shove it towards them and I would explain that you wanted them to write in it. As they opened the pages they would see all the other messages and grasp what to do. You would carry it tight in your hands, your fingers squeezing the cover, the card disintegrating within weeks. I learnt to buy you hard-backed notebooks. Now you have moved on again. Now your favourite things to hold are maps: ordnance survey maps, the pink and the orange ones. I've put up a shelf in your bedroom and the number of maps you've collected is growing. Your favourite maps are north and south Pembrokeshire. There are 204 pink Landranger maps to collect and you've started; you only want ones where people you meet live, or used to live, or places they tell you about. You take a pile of your maps everywhere with you. You hold five, six, seven, eight of them in your hands. They are constantly ripping and tearing; you ask me to sellotape them up. It has become a bedtime routine: I sit on your bed and you pass me the maps that need rescuing. Dotted over these maps are crosses marking places where people you have met actually live. A part of your brain understands: you are your grandfather's grandson; Spike has been drawing maps for years. My good friend Bab's husband John has heard about this and has sent you a bag through the post. It's not any old bag – this is a Czechoslovakian Tank Commander map bag. I am impressed and so are you. It is rectangular and made of brown sturdy leather. You put all your favourite maps inside the bag and hold on to it tight. It goes everywhere with you for a number of years and my sellotaping duties decrease until suddenly the bag is discarded in the future; you are back to holding them loose again.

Today and from now on if we go anywhere you need your maps with you. If I pick you up from school they have to be waiting in the car. They seem to act as a security blanket and a soother; they stop you hitting out – instead you squeeze them tight when you feel anxious. Later you will add an address book to this pile. You will work out that if you get a person's postcode you can find where they live on Google Earth. Later when I enter your bedroom I will find you silent, staring at your computer screen as you drive down roads from here to a new there.

⌣

When the provision of respite eventually comes the silence stuns. One full day and night every fortnight and with it comes guilt that I could not cope.

I stand still in your empty room, my constant activity halted: you have gone. Your suitcase was packed, the items list filled: socks, pants, PJs, dressing gown, trousers, shirt, jumper, tie. Tie? Yes, a tie, you love wearing it. It's for you to chew or else your clothes will be chewed to shreds. Medicine bag, washbag, wheelchair, walking frame, your maps in their plastic case to clutch tightly to take into the shower with you, take into bed.

Just one night. Tomorrow you will be home again.

The house is silent and my mind unravels at what it wants to be able to do but my body will not let it. My body needs to sleep.

I had thought that the respite would release the rest of the family. That we would be able to do 'normal' things for one day a fortnight, take trips out together, visit friends, eat out for a treat. This does happen eventually and the respite is increased to one day a week also but not at first, not for a year at least. Instead Natasha and Jack erupt. They bicker and shout at each other and fight for attention. Then there is door slamming and tears. 'What the hell's up with the kids?' Greg asks. Have we damaged them? Have we traumatised them having to witness all of your needs for so long? They have been waiting in the background for us to be able to give them some time and attention. They must have known there was no point before. Now they shout and cry and we listen, try to make up for all that's gone on.

Much later, when you turn eighteen as I write this story, your brother and sister seem happy and content. Our friends with young children will tell us they want their children to grow up to be like ours. They will comment on how open they are, how kind and caring they are towards you, to little ones, how active and interested in life they seem.

There are no guarantees; I know that things could change in an instant, but at this distant moment in the future as I write I feel some peace and relief. We are getting towards adulthood and we are all still together. They care about you even though you are still annoying Jack with your touching. We are all speaking, joking, laughing somehow.

THIRTEEN

We've moved house down the coastline to a property close to a village where Jack's primary school is. Tasha's about to start secondary school in the town where your special needs school is based. The logistics of getting you all where you needed to be hadn't worked where we were. And Jack had no boys to play with at all in the old village. He'd wander the two streets on his own kicking stones past empty holiday houses, he'd spend hours outside alone just to get away from your noises. Our 'dream' house hadn't worked. You were able to hear every sound through the timber framed walls, you could hear humming sounds and your screams were becoming louder and louder.

We got lucky. A rare house without neighbours had come onto the market and it's perfect for us. The holiday season had just ended and the house price had been crazily slashed by a third. It would have been snapped up immediately if it had come on in the springtime but instead we had a chance to buy it. We borrowed all of my parents' retirement savings (which we eventually managed to repay when the other house that we built was sold) and our offer was accepted. We'd lost the chance of making money through holiday lets but this new house had other potential. Maybe we could set up a campsite in the field that has come with it instead? When word spread that the new house's price had been dropped so dramatically people had clamoured and phoned the owner making cash offers, he told us, but he refused. He said he would wait for us: he wanted children in the village, people living here. What a star, which it turned out he was: he's the local celebrity, a famous ex-rugby player. Our new house will always be known as his. The postman, the deliveryman, even the council will say, 'Ah, you live in Peter Morgan's old house, do you?' When we have a chimney fire next year, even the firemen will ask us which bedroom Peter Morgan had slept in!

At last your sounds are more muted and we all find it easier. Tasha and Jack have bedrooms upstairs away from your squeals. We still have to sleep above you, we can't make either of them do it, but it's not quite as bad. And in your bedroom there's space for a piano, bought by your uncles Peter and John; you can have a commode next to your bed for the toilet at night-time, and your wheelchair can turn around easily in there. And downstairs, but away from your bedroom, there is an open main living and kitchen space through which you can bang your walker up and down, and in which we can talk when you are asleep.

Greg misses the architecture of our old house; I miss the wood, the glass and the light, but it was too remote, it feels better to be a bit closer to life.

And Kevan the builder's face brightens when we introduce him to the new owners of the house that he built. They are wealthy holiday homeowners with lots of work for him to carry out. He'll re-sand and varnish the beaten wood floors and plane down the dented doorframes. He'll upgrade the kitchen and take out the cast iron bath that we'd struggled to get up the stairs. He'll rip up the beautiful oak deck at the back that I loved and he hated, and give it away as firewood and instead put down concrete blocks. He's so pleased to have 'his' house back; he is able to tidy it up.

~

'Why did you do that to me today, Louis?'

Natasha has walked through the front door, dumped her school bag on the floor and continued through the living room into the kitchen, where you are sitting at the table eating your after-school snack. You ignore Natasha and instead stare ahead and lift your spoon heaped high with rice pudding and place it into your mouth and swallow.

'Louis, can you hear me?' Natasha says standing over you.

You stare ahead and ignore her but I detect your body waiting, ears listening for her to continue.

'Louis, why are you ignoring Tasha? What happened, Tasha?' I ask.

'You know what happened, don't you, Louis? Why don't you tell Mum?'

You lift up another spoon. You know we are both watching you and the edges of your lips twitch but you make no attempt to answer.

'Louis!' Natasha says exasperated.

'What happened, Tashi?' I ask.

Tasha has recently started secondary school. It's next to your special needs school and has a large sports field that backs up to your school grounds fence.

'Well, I spotted Louis in his playground. He was sitting in his wheelchair near the fence so I took my new friends over to meet him, didn't I, Louis?'

You stay silent.

'I said, "Hello, Louis, do you want to meet my friends?" And do you know what he did?'

'What did you do?' I ask.

You are grinning a big wide smile. You let out a snort and a laugh, hunch your shoulders and giggle.

'Go on, Louis, tell Mum what you did.'

You are doubled over laughing now.

Natasha gives up trying to make you tell me. She's laughing herself.

'He said, "Who are you?"'

⁓

You are screaming again, painful shrieks, your mouth wide open, your face pink, as the sharp notes escape from your throat, reach every room in the house.

I've become your newest obsession that causes you distress. I've joined the knife and the scissors that you need to be hidden, the blender that must be unplugged, the plastic bags that hurt your ears and the car door that must have the child lock on (you know you will pull the handle, unable to resist that uncontrollable urge).

Not all of your obsessions upset you, some can give you pleasure. Take the zip for example; the soothing sound as the zip slides up and down. It must give you tingles down your spine, caress your ears because you sit there silent and still in your wheelchair with a distant look in your eyes as I zip up my coat or zip up my bag.

But I don't give you pleasure. My very presence has started to cause you distress. My every action, my every word must be seen and heard. You cannot miss a thing or a suffocating panic overwhelms you, leads to desperate screams.

'Mummy, what are you doing?'

'Louis, I'm just trying to make the tea.'

'Mummy, what are you saying?'

'I'm just trying to talk to Dad.'

'Mummy, Mummy, what did you say just then?'

'It is four o'clock in the morning. I was asleep.'

You fight sleep, thrashing in your bed, calling out for me at the slightest sound.

I'm silently weeping. The tears trickle, etching a route down my cheeks, dropping from my jaw.

The front door slams. I slam it with a force that should splinter it to pieces. I stand in the darkness and look at the star-filled sky, the moon, feel the still black night swallow me whole.

When I come inside later my face is swollen and cold.

'He stopped screaming the moment you went out the door, went to sleep within five minutes.'

~

'Where did you go last night, Mummy?'
    'Just out.'
    'Did you go for a bike ride?'
    'Is that what you would like me to have done?'
    'Did you wear your red coat?'
    'Yes.'
    'Did you zip it up?'
    'Yes.'
    'Will you go for a bike ride again tonight?'
    'Yes, Louis, I will.'

I have found a solution. Now I must go for a bike ride every night and at last you will sleep. We were doing well before that operation screwed things up again and sucked us into this Kafkaesque nightmare.

~

I found David by recommendation. I didn't hold out much hope, I had become tainted; but I gave him a call, explained our predicament.

    He said to me gently in his calm way, 'Let me come and see if there is anything I can do to help your son.'

On his first visit he showed me the damage, asking you to lift your foot up and down, to the side, as it hung there unmoving, in its twisted position.

'He cannot move his foot,' he said quietly, 'and no wonder he falls when he tries to stand. His hamstrings are shortened from sitting for so long, his legs cannot straighten.'

So that is why you are unable to lie flat in your bed, sleeping with your legs bent, slumping forwards over them when sleep eventually comes.

You look at David with a face filled with the hope that I have lost, and your words breathe out and burn me.

'You will help me to walk.'

He answers you honestly, 'I will try, Louis, I will try.'

'Just try,' you say back with a lilt to your voice.

~

We are going to see the band Wonderbrass. They are a twenty-five-piece jazz band that play at the Druidstone Hotel every year. It's become a tradition of theirs to come down to this remote part of Wales out of season. The band plays a concert upstairs in the dining room and then stays the night at the hotel for free, jamming down in the bar later well into the early hours. A few guests and locals like us turn up to listen. They're lucky if they manage to have an audience of thirty in the dining room to play to on this Sunday afternoon. We sit around small tables in two thirds of the room and half the band members squeeze into the remaining area while the rest are left lingering in the corridor. As the band starts to play different members come and go through the door to allow others to join in the performance, play a trumpet or trombone solo. You sit in a dining chair in the middle of the room facing the band spellbound.

When they come to the end of a tune you whoop and clap your hands jerkily but when they play you are miraculously silent. This is unheard of for you. Your concentration is normally short-lived; your noises are plentiful at any other type of performance we've ever attended, we often have to leave because of them, but not here.

After the concert I take you up to the lead clarinet player and conductor of the band to buy a CD of their music.

'Louis's your number one fan,' I tell him and you reach out your hand, hold onto the man's hand tight and invite him to our house.

⌒

Bit by bit, over this last year, your hamstrings have been massaged and stretched, your legs gradually straightened, and the pains in your body, your hips, your knees have reduced. And now you are standing up from your wheelchair. Holding tightly onto your frame you slowly rise and sit back down, rise and stand, and today you are lifting each foot off the ground, beaming, counting out loud as you take tiny steps in the air.

My hands are shaking as I hold the digital camera from

a distance to capture this milestone, something to celebrate with all those who love you. Thank goodness we have found David. He is someone at last who knows how to help you, someone who understands.

But just as I discover the best way to help you, I find we are thwarted.

'We do not advise the use of a sports therapist. We strongly advise working under a physiotherapist's instruction. We have serious concerns about what you are doing. You are over-exercising; there is incorrect positioning to Louis's feet.'

David has appeared at our house with a letter in his hand.

'We intend to report Mr Usher to the complaints tribunal at the Chartered Institute of Physiotherapists for misrepresenting himself. This could ultimately be a prisonable offence.'

What offence? They are not happy about the YouTube footage I have posted for family and friends of David teaching Louis to walk. I have called him a sports physiotherapist and it transpires the name physiotherapist is owned by the chartered profession. I can only say he is performing physiotherapy. I change the wording; it is my error, not David's, and I make that known.

You hold the telephone to your ear and listen to glowing praise from your uncle Peter with an enormous smile on your face. When you come off the phone you ask to watch the YouTube footage again. I wheel you over to the computer in the living room and turn on the screen. There you are in your wheelchair wearing a jumper and grey jersey shorts and long black cushioned socks up to your knees. These socks protect your legs against sores from the hard plastic splints you are wearing that attempt to hold your twisted feet flat, and over these are a pair of black leather shoes, oversized in order to fit. Your walking frame is positioned in front and David is crouched down on his knees at your eye level giving you words of encouragement to grip onto your frame, pull yourself up, straighten your body and bend each leg in the air, make stationary steps and count. As we watch the clip to the end we see you sit back in your wheelchair with contentment on your face and I notice your chest is heaving, you are breathing deeply from the exertion of this short physical act.

FOURTEEN

'I want to go up the steps.'

'Yes, Louis, hopefully you will in time.'

I'm pushing you up a ramp into a large warehouse building down by the river in town. Helpfully, there is a small car park off to the left of the building that makes it easy for us to attend David's sports therapy sessions.

'Louis just said that he wants to try the steps outside.'

'That's a good idea, Louis, something to aim for. We'll practise your stepping in here and when you're ready we'll try the steps outside.'

Today you sit on the couch with your legs over the side. You stand and sit, stand and sit. David times how long you can stand before needing to sit back down on the couch. One second, two seconds, three . . .

'Well done, Louis, three seconds. Now we will aim to make it four.'

～

You've had an adventure today. Greg went to Tesco with Tasha and Jack to get Halloween costumes and fake blood and you wanted to go with them too.

I've heard the car arrive back outside on the drive, and Tasha and Jack have burst into the house, through the living room and into the kitchen where I am.

'You won't believe what happened!' Natasha says excitedly.

'What?' I ask.

Greg's wheeling you in through the living room towards us.

'We lost Louis in Tesco,' Jack shouts.

'What! What do you mean you lost Louis?'

'We were looking down the aisle trying to find the fake blood and Dad had left Louis in the wheelchair at the end. When we turned round he'd gone,' Tasha tells me.

'Louis!' I exclaim.

'We were running down all the aisles trying to find him and Dad ran to the shop entrance to ask the security man if he'd seen a boy in a wheelchair leave the store,' Jack says.

'The man said no, he must still be in here,' Greg adds. 'We watched as he used the cameras to look down each of the aisles but Louis wasn't there. So he checked upstairs and when he got to the far end of the shop in the café there he was on the security screen. He was sitting at a table in his wheelchair with a drink.'

I really am amazed.

'Louis, how did you sneak away so quietly?'

'He went up in the lift,' Jack announces.

'Louis! And how did you get a drink?'

'I asked for some water,' you say calmly.

It's as if you've metamorphosed into a different child. We all stare at you. Then you do a few whoops and wave your arms and legs up and down and we relax our gaze. You're back to normal.

242

It is an incredible moment for us as a family. It's the first time you've done anything independently; you've taken us all by surprise. But how did it feel for you? What went on in your mind? You don't let on, you don't say anything else, but you enjoy hearing us tell the story to others.

⁓

You want a tambura for your birthday. I suppose it is easier than the steamroller, escalator, double bass and tuba that you've asked for before. You've already got a euphonium, a guitar, a didgeridoo and still want a sitar. Every year on your birthday or at Christmas these are the things that you'll ask for.

'What's one of those, Louis?'

'And a Tibetan horn,' you throw in as well.

Greg says it will only be a waste of money, that you won't be able to play it, and our friend Squidge tells us he'll adapt an old sitar of his instead.

'That's not a tambura!' you tell me with clear disappointment on your birthday. 'This is a tambura.' And you show me on YouTube on your computer. The woman holds the neck of a large Indian instrument, speaks with a soft American accent as she twangs. It is repetitive and mesmerising. Where will I find one of those?

But I manage. Miraculously, I find one for Christmas and now an enormous black case sits in your room. And you love it. You proudly show anyone who visits. At bedtime you ask

Greg to tune it. I hear droning drifting out of your room and Greg calling out my name softly to come and see.

'Look at Louis.'

You sit upright in your bed with your pyjama top in your mouth and your head nodding forwards, your eyes rolling back; it has sent you into a trance. And we use it now to help to soothe you at bedtime, calm you, send you to sleep.

⌒

I take you out of school early and drive you across town to the swimming pool. I've found Sue who is going to try to help you. It's taken a bit of negotiation with the local council to allow it to occur – 'it's not in our policy document' – and the pool is fully booked after school hours for clubs and children's swimming lessons. There's nothing for disabled children after school, not those who would require one to one assistance. They tell me there is no demand. But I demand repeatedly so now I've managed to secure a session as long as it happens before school time ends.

The disabled changing room makes an enormous difference when taking you there. I dread turning the corner towards the room in case I see a light on under its door. Then we will have to wait outside as you yell and cry that you will be late for your lesson.

You pull at your shirt buttons as I help you take off your school clothes. You can't wait. I get you into the metal chair on wheels and wheel you through the communal area past the showers and out onto the poolside. The chair makes a creaking screeching sound as I push and you join in. Little children clutch their parents' legs with fingers in their ears as we pass. The winch has been put into place and your metal seat is clipped onto the hoist frame, like a mini crane; it lifts you into the air and swings you down into the water. I can't help but notice how badly twisted your feet look as they shake up and down with excitement.

The leisure centre is newly built and the main pool is split into two sections. One is deep at both ends and limited to lane swimming; the other is designed to be flexible, its floor height can be altered. It's an amazing facility to have on our doorstep, and now that your lessons have started to be weekly the pool staff are getting to know you. They've all smiled and agreed to be your friend on Facebook as they pump the hoist, and raise you into the air.

Today Tom, the lifeguard, has already changed the height of the floor to allow you to stand in the water and Sue is walking you up and down the pool over and over.

It is helping you to be upright, helping you to exercise your legs, helping bit by bit to strengthen you.

I would never guess that in four years' time you would be swimming. You will still swallow buckets of water, retch so loudly that people will leave the pool, but you will glide by and your legs will sway behind like a tail as you swim the length of the pool eight times in a row as Sue wades in the water beside you, rushes to place her hand on the end wall to cushion your head as you swim into it hard.

⌣

You are shrieking. The sound is swirling around the living room. Your arms are raised up towards your shoulders, elbows bent, hands cupped and fingers curled like claws. Your mouth is stretched across your face in an enormous smile. The clunking sound of your frame has ceased; you've abandoned it at the end of the room. Instead the warm thud of footsteps is resounding off the wooden boards as you balance towards me, wobbling with each step. I am calling out to you, telling you to keep going.

'Louis, you're nearly there. You can do it, Louis, you can do it.'

⌣

Along with your exercises with David another miracle has occurred. We've found something that can occupy you. Something you can concentrate on all by yourself and enjoy. Who would have thought it was possible? It's taken a while, four years, for your brain to make the full connection you need to be able to do it: you can play the piano.

It was Emma who suggested it. I met her at your school when you were ten. She is a parent of a disabled child who goes to your school; her son Jack is older than you. Her

Jack came over and held Natasha's nose tight when we'd come to collect you from school one day. Emma had walked quickly up to us and apologised, had asked Jack to stop immediately. Little Tasha had stood motionless. Our eyes had been locked on each other. I'd been smiling reassuringly as Emma had got Jack to let go of her nose.

'Well done, sweetheart,' I whispered to Tasha. 'You handled that really well.' I squeezed her hand and put my arm around her. Emma started to talk. She revealed she was a music teacher and in particular she taught piano.

'Ah, I'd really love my children to learn the piano.'

'Would you like me to try all three?'

'Yes, I would.' I was thrilled as I agreed.

'It never worked with our Jack. We could try with Louis but I've no idea if it will work or not, but shall we give it a go?'

So we did.

At the start you just sat there on the piano chair with your head bowed and listened as Emma played a tune and then sang to you. She placed the music onto the stand and traced the notes with her finger calling out the letters as she played. It took over a year for you to respond and play a few simple notes and then another year before it seemed to click in your brain.

'I don't really understand what is happening with Louis,' Emma told me. 'If you watch he turns the pages at the right place in the music but he's not looking up, he's looking down at the keys. I think he is learning the tune off by heart, by ear.'

And so you are. You hold your fingers above the keys and press gently. Even though your playing is filled with mistakes, it has a sensibility that takes all of us by surprise. Your fingers are stiff and crooked; you can barely hold a pen. You cannot write except crudely your name, L – o – u – i – s, like the first scrawls of a three year old, yet here, remarkably, you are playing a tune. And you won't miss a lesson even though the others have long since given up. Emma beams at the door.

'Ah, here's my favourite pupil.'

We increase your lesson to an hour and you still want to stay for longer.

'I have to be careful,' Emma tells me. 'If I play or sing a wrong note he remembers and copies me.'

And for the first time in the fourteen years of your life you have something to do. You've not been able to do anything yourself before this. Take reading, for example: you can read words but you don't understand a story. You don't seem to be able to differentiate between fact and fiction. The other day you asked me, 'Where does Little Bo Peep live?' You can't follow a film either, but you can listen to music. It must require a different part of your brain, a different kind of understanding.

You become spellbound, mesmerised, as Emma plays and then you sit in your seat and lift your hands and respond. Your fingers hamper the way that you touch the keys but you overcome this. You use the sides of your little finger, play as if you have claws that can bend and we listen. The music comes from the piano in your bedroom and floats around the house, up to our bedroom above. And it calms you and it calms us. It sends us all to a place of peace for a while.

FIFTEEN

Jack's taken up surfing and it's difficult to watch him down on the beach and care for you too, and the thing with surfing is it takes quite a long time in the water.

Jack's been having surf lessons on a Tuesday with his friend Jamie and Jamie's dad Mike takes them both to their lesson. I feel grateful, guilty and torn. I want to be doing these parent things too but I can't. I have to rely on the kindness of others in order for Jack and Natasha not to miss out. Tonight it is Thursday and Jack is excited – 'surf is up' – but there is no one who can take him down to the beach except you and me. The frustration of always saying 'I'm afraid I can't, Jack' gets to me this time, it hurts, and I say, 'Yes, okay,' and I get you ready and take you both down in the car. Jack's already in his wetsuit and jumps out as soon as we get there; he grabs his board and is running towards the beach and the waves. Before he is out of earshot I call out.

'I'll be watching you from the car, Jack. Be careful, and don't be too long.'

It's too cold for you to be wheeled down onto the beach in this wind. We sit in the car on the road looking out at the sea and a tiny black shape in the waves. There isn't anyone else in the sea tonight; it's out of season, an autumn school night. The light is fading, turning to dusk, and Jack's shape is getting harder for me to pick out and then all of a sudden he's gone, I can't see him. I'm out of the car.

'Louis, you will have to wait here on your own. I need to check Jack,' and I lock you in.

I'm running down the beach calling Jack's name, looking out in vain into the sea. The waves seem to have grown bigger even though the tide's receding and then as I reach the water's edge I see his small dark shape in the foam and I wave frantically at him to come in and the relief is enormous that he's all right.

Jack catches the next wave in towards me as I wait on the sand. He stands happily and starts instantly to tell me about the waves he has caught.

'Did you see me catch that last big one, Mum?' he asks as we walk across the beach back to the car. I don't want to spoil this moment by telling him how worried I was and I squash away my anxieties about you alone in the car. Instead I embrace this feeling of closeness as we cross the expanse of silvered sand in the dusk. You are fine when we get back to the car, you aren't troubled at all, so I've managed precariously to balance the needs of you both, and for once help Jack do something he loves.

⌒

You've never had a friend, but today you come home from school and tell me you have one.

'Can Oonagh come for a sleepover?'

'Who's Oonagh, Louis?'

'She's my friend.'

'Is she one of the teachers or assistants?'

'She's in my class.'

'Hey, that's exciting.'

'Can she come for a sleepover?'

'Well, it's probably best if she comes over to play first.'

'I want her to come for a sleepover.'

Oonagh writes you a letter. You unzip your school bag and pull out the envelope and ask me to read it.

I stare at the letters written in pencil. They are small and square and make no sense. Then I realise that most of the letters are upside down and back to front.

I am sorry Louie I can not come for a sleepover at your howse please stop asking me.

'Can Oonagh come for a sleepover?'

'No, Louis, she can't. But we could see if she is allowed to come to play here sometime. Maybe over half-term?'

'Will you ask Oonagh's mummy? Will you ask Oonagh's mummy?' you repeatedly ask me all evening.

'Let's write a letter, you can take it to school.'

You whoop.

I carefully write a letter to Oonagh and her parents and ask if she would like to come over to play, I invite them as well. I say we can accommodate whatever best suits them and give my telephone number. I put the letter in an envelope and put it in the schoolbook with a note asking the teacher to give the letter to Oonagh.

We don't hear anything for a while and then I get a phone call. Oonagh's mother is fine about our invitation. Just Oonagh will come; we are going to meet halfway to lessen the journey.

When I come later to collect you from school for swimming you greet me with your favourite question, 'Have you heard from Oonagh's mummy?'

'You'll be so lucky,' Mr Moon, your support assistant, mutters. He's usually jolly so I'm puzzled.

I look down at you in your walking frame. You are leaning forwards as you try to stand still.

'Yes, Louis,' I grin. 'I have, and she can. She can come next Thursday for the day.'

It went wrong, though, didn't it?

At first it was fine. The changeover worked and her mother was friendly. I can well understand she'd be uneasy to send her daughter off somewhere new. Oonagh was nervous; she replied to every repetitive question you asked with a 'no' as she nervously moved her feet. Greg and I asked friendly questions and offered nice treats and then you played a game of 'Guess Who'. Well, Oonagh played but you couldn't concentrate, could you? You seemed overcome with excitement at her being here. You showed her your favourite things in your bedroom, your piano, euphonium and guitar, your CDs and laptop too.

'Will you be my friend on Facebook?' you asked.

'No, Louis, I can't.'

'Go on,' you giggled.

'No, you mustn't ask.'

'Louis, it's rude to giggle.'

You loved every minute and Oonagh seemed happy that you found her funny even though she told you off. But she flushed bright pink when you asked her about Facebook again. You suggested I ask her mum.

'Oh no, don't do that.'

I left you two playing and went upstairs to get a book from my room. I heard Oonagh's footsteps go into the bathroom and the door close; I heard your footsteps following. You were giggling as I ran down the stairs fast. You were pushing the bathroom door.

'No, Louis!'

I grabbed the door handle and pulled it closed quickly.

'Louis, don't do that. It's not polite.'

'It's rude,' you said with a look of delight.

'I'm so sorry, Oonagh,' I said when she came out. 'That was an accident.'

You come home from school howling. I take your arm and help you out of the bus and inside where you sit in your wheelchair in your bedroom and cry. Tears run down your cheeks and drop into your lap.

'Oonagh says she can never come to my house again.'

'Oonagh says her mummy says I'm a rude boy.'

'Oonagh says never ever.'

'Can Oonagh come again, Mummy? Can she come again? I won't do it again.'

I go to your school and ask to have a private word with your teacher.

'How is Louis at school with Oonagh? Is Oonagh okay with him? He's very upset right now.'

The teacher says that the two of you ask especially to sit and do things together. She doesn't think you are bothering Oonagh. She says you both appear happy.

I write a second letter. I've tried calling but had no answer. I explain that the opening of the toilet door was an innocent accident, that I am sorry and that I should have explained in more detail at the time.

I tell you I've written a letter and we will have to wait and see. You ask me if I've heard every day. You cry in your room every night. We hear nothing for a very long time. So long that I think we never will. Then a letter comes back. It is kind but clear.

'Louis does not understand "no" and this upsets Oonagh. I hope that you understand that Louis would be better choosing a different play date. We hope you understand and wish you the very best for the future.'

I carefully choose a time to tell you the answer and you open your mouth and wail. You say Oonagh's name. You pleadingly ask, 'Why can't she come here again?'

*

It takes a long while for you to accept but eventually you stop asking me to try. Today I hear you singing her name. I hear your voice break into a song. You sing a short phrase to yourself as you sit in your bedroom alone.

'Oonagh? Yes, Louis. Oonagh? Yes, Louis.'

You sing it joyfully, today, tomorrow, the next day, over and over again.

⌣

We need to go to Edinburgh but you don't like going any-where for more than a day. You haven't stayed away overnight for years, not since our trip to London. It was the disastrous trip to Holland that started it; we have been struggling with getting you to travel again ever since.

We'd thought that a trip to Holland was a good idea. I remember the excitement in the build-up. We were going on a summer holiday abroad. We were going to do something 'normal' like other families do. It never occurred to us you would not comply. On that trip you managed to cry for a full six days. Our marriage was at the point of breaking.

We'd thought carefully about how to have a good time with you and Tasha and Jack. We'd chosen Holland because it was flat, and had booked a holiday park with bikes and a pull-along bubblecar for you. There were forests and a pool. Tasha and Jack were beyond excited about the idea. It had still been a daunting prospect, with your toileting, feeding and physical care, but we had thought it would work.

As the plane rumbled down the runway you had begun to scream and you kept it up. It hadn't occurred to any of us that you wouldn't be able to travel.

At the holiday park you asked, 'What is a holiday?'

'It's meant to be fun, Louis. We explore, enjoy the sunshine, go for rides, see new things, go to the pool, relax.'

'I don't like holidays. I want to go home.'

And so it persisted. All you wanted to do was watch CBeebies, which didn't exist in Holland.

Greg went into shutdown. He could not cope any more with the screaming and became silent and I found myself like a single parent taking you all down to the pool. Tasha and Jack were happy using the water slides and Randy, the pool attendant, saved the day. He gave you lots of attention, helped to carry you up the steps of the slide as I caught you down below, but God it was hard.

'Never again,' we had said when we got back and it's become a family joke that you don't like Holland. You call the Dutch 'Ditch people' and like to scream when Greg plays 'the holiday game':

'Hey Louis, why don't we go on a little holiday?'

'Nooo!' Screams.

'Ah come on, Louis. Let's go to Holland.'

'Nooo!' You scream louder, 'I don't like Ditch people!'

'But Louis, it will be fun.'

'No, no, no!' Screams.

'Okay, let's stay at home then.'

You erupt into giggles at the kitchen table.

And now we need to go to Edinburgh.

You've been screaming loudly about not wanting to go, but we haven't got any choice. We need to fly up the night before to be there first thing in the morning for an assessment and then come straight back home.

'We are going to have to stay somewhere, Louis, but it will be fun. You'll have me and Dad with you.'

You continue screaming loudly.

'How about bagpipes! You'll get to see some of those when we go up.'

This takes you a while to process. You stop screaming. You look thoughtful. There's a very long pause. You stuff your tie into your mouth and give it a chew and then you pull it out with one of your hands. You drop your maps and both of your arms start to wave up and down in the air and whack onto the kitchen table, your voice making whooping guttural sounds and your legs join in kicking under the table. You are so excited you can't control your body actions.

'I want to see bagpipes.'

I've found an apartment with kitchen facilities close to Princes Street for the night on special offer. I find people to have Tasha and Jack overnight and we are off on the journey to Bristol airport. As we pick up our tickets, you look up from your wheelchair and tell the tall man behind the counter that you are scared. He answers you with a deep Scottish accent.

'Och don't be scared, you'll have fun,' he says with a big smile, and you grin back at him with the tie still stuffed in your mouth. I can tell that you like him; you like friendly men with a sense of humour.

Your habit of touching people inappropriately in the groin has been increasing recently. This latest compulsion is a disaster to manage and makes it difficult to take you any-where near other people. The more we mention not doing it the more you do, so we have to ignore your actions. I'll say, 'Touch your bracelet, Louis,' (I've put a knotted cord around your wrist for this) and at the same time I'll try to distract you. 'Oh, look over there at that, Louis.' You don't realise how serious this latest compulsion is. It's been creeping up for years, just an arm outstretched so people moved their bodies away, but now it's a full-blown swipe. Initially I think you liked how the touching made people jump. It would make you laugh the same way that you laugh at Mr Bean. But now you are compelled to take a quick swipe at people's groins every time. It makes them jump back, gives them a shocked and embarrassed look and you think it is funny.

'No, no, Louis, it is not funny, it is very, very serious.'

'It is rude,' you say with obvious delight.

You are at whatever the developmental stage is for taking delight in rude things but the problem is you are older and therefore it is treated much more seriously. Your school has begun filling in 'incident' forms whenever you take a swipe at another child or member of staff; they've been teaching you it's 'not appropriate'. And you howl now because you don't want to be near enough to touch anyone. You don't want to be 'naughty'. It's so complex to manage how best to cope.

We are going through security. I have to push you through the metal detector screen in your chair and the alarm goes off.

'Please can you go back and go through on your own?' I am asked.

I pass back through and the alarm is silent.

'I'm afraid I'll have to do a quick check of your boy,' says the security man. He rummages behind your back, along up your legs and swiftly across your groin.

'That was rude, Mummy!' you say with a wide smile. 'That was inappropriate!'

We use the airport's disabled service, which requires us to wait while everyone else boards the plane first. You sit patiently in your wheelchair holding your maps tight and chewing your tie. The lift takes us up to the front door of the plane. We abandon the wheelchair and Greg and I step-walk you into the aircraft. The flight is full. People look up and watch us approaching, we are a few rows in; children stare, others look away not wanting to appear rude. I'm trying to balance you and stop you falling over. I'm also aware that you might try to touch someone. The flight attendant smiles.

'Are you okay there?'

She has bleached blond hair and orange foundation on her face. She is wearing a tight fitting grey pencil skirt and black high heels.

'Hello, I'm Louis, nice to meet you,' you say and hold out your hand. She shakes it and you hold on tight. You don't let go but grip her hand hard. She keeps smiling. I'm impressed. She's professional.

'Are you on Facebook?' you ask her.

'Yes, I am.'

'Will you be my friend?'

'Of course, Louis, of course.'

Greg's getting flustered. 'Come on, Louis, let go of the lady's hand.'

You let go after a bit of tugging by me and we manage to get down the aisle to our seats.

Phew, we've survived the first part of this journey. Oh no, bloody hell. In the three seats in front are three heads poking above the head rests and the middle one is bald and shiny. Your arm is out and you've managed to touch it before I have time to grab your hand. The man jerks and turns slightly.

'I'm so sorry,' I say quickly. 'No, Louis, don't.'

Greg hisses with rage, 'Louis, stop it.'

I hold onto your hand tightly. Your other arm is lifting and Greg's grabbed it. We are both sitting there holding your arms, linking ours through your own. Your body jolts as each arm compulsively lifts and one of us manages to hold it back. Greg is sweating; he is beetroot. 'Stop it, Louis,' he whispers into your ear but you can't, you just can't stop yourself.

The plane is taxiing down the runway.

'When we take off I'll swap seats,' I say. 'I'll put Louis on the aisle seat.' At least then it won't be shining in front of you.

We swap with difficulty and I hold your left arm. From your new seat you make a half-hearted attempt to stretch your right arm to touch the bald man's head.

'I can't reach,' you say.

'No, you can't; you can't reach him now,' I whisper.

You can reach if you really tried. We both know it but if we pretend, it works. You look across the aisle and start stretching out your arm but you keep it bent.

'I can't reach there either.'

'No, you can't.'

You start to relax a little. You grab your maps off your lap and hold them tight, chew your tie. You are quiet. I hold your left arm tight and feel the urge like an electric shock run through you over and over as your arm tries to rise and is stopped. In time your urge reduces. Halfway through the flight I can feel myself relax your arm hold a little, you've settled at last. Greg has shut his eyes; his head is against the window. We knew this journey was going to be an ordeal; we know we have to get through this somehow for your sake.

The flight attendant is coming down the aisle with drinks. She is passing us by. I notice you looking. You look over towards Greg, his eyes are closed; you look back to the aisle, back towards Greg then very quickly you reach out your right arm and quickly touch the flight attendant's bottom. She gives no reaction, makes no sign it happened.

We have made it. I am pushing you up the hill from the airport bus stop at Waverley Station towards Princes Street.

Where are the damn bagpipes? Usually there's a piper on the corner but this evening there is no one. You are getting anxious.

'I want to go home.'

'It's fine, Louis. Just one night and then you'll be home.'

And then I hear the distant whine of the pipes coming in the direction of Princes Street towards our apartment. You start to help with the wheels, pushing them in excitement. We reach the top of the hill and I see a short man with dark hair, a very round belly and a green tartan kilt; he's filling his cheeks with air. I push you across the road as Greg pulls our bag behind. You are pushing the wheels of the chair with a force I've not felt before. You break away. I'm running, and shouting, 'Louis watch out!' A woman jumps out of the way as you head straight for the piper. I grab the handles just as you slam on your brakes to stop dead beside him. The piper stops playing.

'Hello, I'm Louis.'

'Hi, Louis, I'm Rocco.'

'Will you play "The Flower of Scotland" for me, Rocco?'

'Sure I will, Louis.'

What were the chances of that? That Rocco would be positioned directly across the road from our apartment? His music follows us into the building and we open the window so you can hear him until he stops. We get through the night with you waking and needing help to the toilet twice. You thrash in your bed and hit your head against the headboard. I pile the pillows up high behind you to try to help, and the

266

staff downstairs upgrade us all for no extra charge, say there is a bigger room we can have. The kitchenette is perfect: we can prepare your food, mash it and feed you without the stress of finding something you can eat that is runny enough for you to swallow.

The next day the assessment is over by lunchtime and Greg and I have a plan to surprise you. Before going back to the airport we push you over to Haymarket Station. Across the road from the railway entrance is a shop that makes its own bagpipes. In the shop we buy you a set of Highland pipes to take home. The bag is made of synthetic material that makes it cheaper, but they sound the same and are easy to play. You've been asking for bagpipes for years and now you have got some. You know you won't be able to play them but you want Greg to do it for you.

Greg has a go in the shop. He blows down the chanter and fills the bag, pumps his arm up and down and it begins to drone, so he moves his fingers. It sounds impressive, bagpipes with a touch of the Eastern.

Your arms flail about in the air and your voice makes guttural sounds of excitement.

So we survive the trip to Scotland. It was even a success of sorts; it certainly beat Holland, that's for sure. Once we get home and are somewhat recovered I ask at the kitchen table over breakfast, 'Hey Louis, that trip wasn't so bad now, was it?'

'I didn't like it.'

'But Louis, you met Rocco, you got some bagpipes.'

'I didn't like it at all,' you say firmly.

I bend over and rest my elbows on the wooden table; I'm at eye level with you. I ask in an inquisitive voice, 'Do you think that maybe sometime we could all go on another trip?'

You start screaming immediately.

⌣

David is carefully step-walking you outside the warehouse. You hold the handrail on one side and David holds your arm on the other as you slowly make your way down the ramp. At the bottom David turns his body towards the three steps but you don't move. You stand still, holding the rail tightly, wobbling.

'Shall we try the three steps then, Louis?'

'No.'

'But I thought you wanted to try the steps?'

'Not those steps.'

You have lifted your head slightly and are looking across the car park past the Bristol Trader pub and over the road towards the tree- and scrub-covered embankment. I've never given that area a glance. We all look. There, cut out of the steep rock face, are lots of concrete steps with handrails and resting platforms and benches. It is an ugly sight. The handrails look dirty and cold, the concrete is rough and stained, the first wooden bench looks rotten. *How have I never noticed those and where do they go?* The steps rise up into woodland. There are over one hundred in view. I will come to discover from you counting them one day in the future, one day when eventually you precariously manage to reach the top with David, that there are 155.

'I want to go up there.'

We laugh incredulously. David answers.

'Well, Louis, that may take a little while longer before you are ready. But it is something to aim for in time.'

You drop your head and I hear you say quietly, 'Just try.'

~

It's David's birthday tomorrow. During your physio session you ask him a question out of the blue.

'How old will you be?'

'I'll be forty-nine, Louis, I'll be forty-nine.'

'Oh, you are getting old.'

'Well, what about the big five-oh next year then, Louis, how about that?'

'You'll be dead soon,' you reply.

~

'You're between a rock and a hard place.'

Mr Monsam is sitting back in his swivel chair and moving it from side to side as he speaks. He has a busy air about him. He's studied you quickly and carefully and is wasting no time in telling us his thoughts. I can tell he has a limited amount of time to spend on us; I can tell he's been working all day; I can tell this is probably the case for him day after day. I am putting your long socks back on, gently trying to get you to relax your foot, to twist it straight and edge it into the splint. Eventually it's on and I am able to slip an enlarged shoe over the top.

'I can see that the surgery has had a negative impact but you're managing to rectify it as best you can. As a surgeon it can be better to keep away at times. In Louis's case if I did anything further he could end up in a wheelchair permanently. We have to face that he is likely to deteriorate over time but this is better than risking forcing him into a chair right now.'

He pauses.

'I wish all of my patients were like you,' he says to you with a smile. 'Louis, you have fine thigh muscles and a strong upper body. Your exercise programme is excellent. Walking and swimming are two forms of exercise I can't recommend enough.'

'This is partly why we have come. Our local physiotherapist is concerned we are over-exercising Louis.'

'I beg your pardon? You can't over-exercise. Louis will let you know if he wants to stop. I think your biggest concern is his skin right now. It is breaking down from the splints rubbing. If this continues he will not be able to walk at all due to the risk of infection and pain.'

'Well, this is it, the splints are meant to help Louis's incorrect positioning but they hurt him. They are concerned we might be damaging his joints through the exercise.'

'Well, it's either that or he's in the wheelchair permanently from now. Where's the logic in that?'

'What do you suggest that we do?'

Mr Monsam ponders a short while.

'I think the splints should be discontinued. I'm not allowed to say the brand of boot in the letter but I suggest you try Dr Martens boots. They will be able to offer Louis flexible support without the fixed structure of the splint. And you'll look cool, Louis, too.'

I feel incredulous. I'd never thought of this as a possibility. I feel an enormous sense of relief; thank goodness I've found this doctor, he seems very experienced.

Mr Monsam lifts his Dictaphone up to his mouth. You double over in giggles as you listen to him speak.

We leave the hospital and go straight to a Dr Martens shop in the centre of Bristol, where we buy you a pair of boots. You try them on in the shop, stand and balance across the room. We can't wait to get home to try them properly.

In the car on the way home you play a game with Greg. You call out from your seat in the back.

'Hello, Mr Monsam.'

Greg lifts his hand to his mouth and pretends he is speaking into a Dictaphone addressing the secretary.

'I inspected Louis White with his parents today full stop.

They explained there are concerns about his splints, sores and the question of over-exercising full stop. I can clarify that Louis White's current exercise programme is imperative to his well-being full stop. Err, let me rewind that a little . . . I suggest a flexible leather boot with lacing, to replace his current splints full stop. I will review again in three months' time with the view to considering Botox injections in the future full stop.'

We email a photograph of you to Mr Monsam's secretary. You are wearing your orange puffy winter coat and have gloves pulled onto your hands. It was cold that December day but the sun was bright. It was a perfect day to go down to the beach to practise your walking on the hard golden sand. I've taken your two hands and helped to tug and pull you out of the chair. Your body is bent and you straighten up uneasily, your feet are hidden but I know they are twisting inside your boots, but the soles look flattish on the sand. You make tiny steps to keep stationary and then I let go. You walk away squealing. Greg snaps the photograph as you come towards him, capturing the joy on your face, your new black laced-up Dr Martens boots.

Greg is my Peter Sellers; he's funny, creative and complex, and his presence livens up our family, helps to make some days become lighter. His gift of laughter in most circumstances makes me think of a Gulag story I once read: men were packed into trains heading across Siberia; they were starving and dying along the way. It was the funny men who were the heroes, the author wrote. It was they who saved the others on that journey to hell, who kept up their spirits, even though there was nothing to hope for, had them laughing together, forming close bonds as they swayed.

And I've noticed you appreciate humour too; you've recognised Greg's and tapped into it. Take today; you're sitting in your wheelchair at the kitchen table eating four Weetabix, mashed up with warm milk, swallowing without a chew.

'I don't like Phil Kay.'

'Hey Louis, do you remember him? That's a long time ago. You were only little, maybe five, when you last saw him,' I respond.

Years ago Phil would pop around to our flat sometimes.

'Hi guys, how are you getting on? How's our wee Louis doing?'

And you would throw yourself backwards onto the floor and thrash around. Phil, with his tangled hair and expressive arm gestures, would look bemused; he was used to being found charming, and I'd steer him out of the living room away from you, instinctively knowing you found him frightening. It's probably his energetic manner I'd always thought, although you could not tell me.

'You remember Phil?' I ask again now.

A high-pitched scream erupts from your mouth. 'I didn't like him.'

'You couldn't speak then; you couldn't tell us.'

'I don't like Phil Kay.'

'But Louis, you like everyone.'

'Not Phil Kay.'

'Why not?'

There is a long pause, long enough to think you will not answer, then without looking up from your breakfast you speak with a smile on your lips.

'I don't know.'

You've gone silent, concentrating on lifting large spoonfuls of Weetabix into your mouth. I begin clattering around in the kitchen as I hear you speak again in a giggling voice.

'Hello, Phil Kay.'

I hear a rustle of paper, Greg clear his throat.

'Hello, Louis,' he says. He draws out the 'hello' and almost shouts out the 'Louis'. It is as if Phil has entered the room.

'Go away, Phil Kay, I do not like you.'

'Och come on now, Louis, surely you must like me?'

Greg raises the word 'me' to a higher pitch. Screams erupt from your mouth.

'Go away, go away.'

'Knock, knock, knock.'

The kitchen table thuds as Greg speaks.

'Who's this knocking at the door? Why it's your good friend . . .'

'Stuart,' you shout out quickly.

'No, it's not Stuart, Louis, good try. It's your good friend
. . .'

'Callum.'

You are starting to shake.

'Och no, Louis, not Callum, it can only be . . . Ph Ph Ph
Ph . . .'

Screams erupt that turn into uncontrollable laughter.

'Stop!' I call out, laughing. 'The noise, it's hurting my ears!'

You enjoy screaming you don't like Phil Kay so much that
you want to play the role game again and again in the kitch-
en and we start to call it your drama therapy.

The first day you meet Colin, you have a surprise. The Phil
Kay game has got out of control. Now everywhere we go and
everyone you meet is greeted with a scream and a garbled
line, 'Go away, Phil Kay, I don't like you.' And you grin at
them wide. Of course no one understands what on earth you
are saying. You love to listen as I try to explain in the supermarket, on the street. But the day that Colin walks through
our front door it is different.

Colin strides in to meet Greg; they met recently when
Greg composed some music for Colin's zoo television programme. Colin could not be more alpha male, he's a wild
Glaswegian in Wales and I know that you'll love him, spot
his accent as soon as you hear his voice.

'Louis, this is Colin,' Greg says to you.

'Nice to meet you, Louis,' Colin shouts.

And you scream at the top of your voice, 'Go away, go away, Phil Kay, I don't like you at all.'

And Colin hears you, hears every word. He towers above you and answers in his strong Glaswegian accent in a clear loud voice.

'No, Louis, I agree with you there. I don't like Phil Kay either.'

You are astounded. You are staring at him with your mouth wide open.

'You're dead right there. Phil Kay? That man is a pain in the ass.'

The 'ass' comes out with a sharp 'a' and a hiss. And that's done it. *Oh no!* There's another expression that you take and savour and repeat over and over.

'Phil Kay, he's a pain in the ass.'

⁓

Your lip is jutted forwards and lowered. You are lying in your bed clutching your maps. I'd heard shouting, heard Greg say something about you having his phone again, and the bedroom door closed firmly. I've come down to check what is wrong.

'I've been naughty. I took Daddy's phone.'

'Don't worry, it's okay.'

'I rang Colin; it's his birthday tomorrow. Can I ring him?'

'Yes, of course you can.'

Colin will get a birthday song early tomorrow. Colin will get a birthday song every year of his life unless he changes his number. You do this to everyone who knows you; you sing them a birthday song first thing in the morning on the day of their birthday. You remember the date when you ask them and then pass over your address book, ask them to write down their phone number for you to call them up when the day comes. Sometimes you have two or three people to call on one morning; I don't know how you remember all these dates, but it's very endearing.

'I rang someone else too.'

'Who did you ring?'

'I rang Phil Kay.'

'Oh, Louis, you didn't!'

'I did.'

We haven't spoken to Phil for years.

'Did he answer?'

'Yes.'

'What did you say?'

I don't really need to ask this, do I?

'"I don't like you."'

'And then what?'

'Stop. Stop asking me questions.'

You're shaking.

'It's okay, don't worry.'

I'm suddenly struck – we were having a long conversation. This is new, it hasn't happened before.

'Will Father Christmas still come? Will I still get lots of presents? Have I been a bad boy?'

You can't understand Father Christmas is not real. I've tried to tell you gently but you can't comprehend this. You're fifteen years old and as excited as a five year old about Christmas coming.

'It's okay, Louis, don't worry, but it's not nice to tell someone you don't like them. It's not kind.'

'I don't like him.'

'Yes, I know, but you don't really know him any more and you don't need to tell him that.'

'I've been naughty, haven't I?'

'Well, try not to do it again. You must stop taking our phones without us knowing and ringing people.'

'Are you going for a bike ride?'

'Yes, Louis, I am. Goodnight, see you in the morning.'

You give me your maps that you are clutching tightly. You know you will wake if they fall off your bed in the night. Our routine is working. I go out of the bedroom and gently close the door. I no longer have to zip my coat up and down a number of times for you to hear in the hall. I don't even have to go out of the front door into the blowing gales and rain to sneak back in. Now I can stand silently in the hall for a few seconds, then slam the front door and edge the living room door open so I can creep in. I hear happy whoops from your room as I complete my manoeuvre holding my breath. Greg is lying on the sofa watching the telly.

'Louis got my phone tonight,' Greg says over the sound of the news.

'I know.'

'He seems to have rung Phil Kay. It says the call was two minutes long so I think he may have left him a message.'

I savour the few seconds before I respond. I try to keep my face blank, stop my mouth from curling, then I can't hold back any longer.

'Phil answered. Lou spoke to him.'

Greg sits bolt upright from his slumped position.

'Oh no, what did he say?'

I laugh. 'I think you can guess.'

⌢

I am sitting on a bench eating a cream scone in the garden of the Druidstone Hotel and you are scooping up ice cream from a bowl. The hotel is perched on the edge of a cliff and our picnic bench is behind a high weathered stone wall. I look around the flowered garden and feel exhaustion and elation at the same time. I cannot believe we have come so far. The word had got out: Louis was attempting to walk all the way from Broadhaven to the Druidstone along the coastal path. When Jane the owner had heard the news she asked Johnny the chef to bake some scones and she greeted us with this surprise.

It was all your idea.

You'd cried a few years ago when some friends of ours had offered to drive you home from the Dru so that Greg and I could have an hour to ourselves walking back along the coastal path. 'I want to come too, I want to come too,' you'd cried out from your wheelchair and I'd had to tell you it was just not possible. So you'd told David that you wanted to walk to the Druidstone. In his usual measured way he'd said you could try it in time.

Over the last year you've been trying out sections of the path with the walking frame; we sourced all-terrain pram wheels and attached them to the legs of your walker to help you get over the rough ground. And today the sweat dripped off your face, your shirt was damp and your tie in shreds. At each bench you sat down with David and he gave you a quiet pep talk. You looked just like a coach and an athlete as you listened to him, I thought. Then you'd awkwardly rise, hold onto the frame and go a little bit further. The walk was two miles long and it's taken you six hours to get here. Ten of us joined you and David and helped to lift the walking frame in places, helped to take both your arms and balance you through narrow sections of the path. Today you have proved to us all that if we just try we can sometimes achieve our dreams.

SIXTEEN

You fell off your walking frame today. You've been getting so strong with your swimming, your exercises with David, that you've started hopping onto the back of your frame and back down. You push your hands on the handle grips and straighten your arms, raise your body up like a gymnast and swing your legs forwards as your bottom rests onto the back of the frame and then you slip quickly back down. It must feel releasing to have this new ability but it's dangerous so we warn you not to, so of course you do it more, it's become a compulsion.

Your jump comes with no warning and you do it at the most precarious of angles and moments when we are taking you from one place to another. And now you have fallen at school. The frame lifted up and flipped backwards and you landed hard on your back and screamed.

You've not hurt yourself badly; it's just a graze and some bruising but it's given you a shock and you are refusing to use the walker now. You howl at school and demand your wheelchair. The school has asked for your chair to be sent in every day and now I'm worried.

We have a meeting.

'If we allow Louis to be in his wheelchair all day at school it will be disastrous for his walking.'

'But he's in danger. It's become a serious health and safety issue, Mrs White.'

'But he needs to walk for his health.'

'Well, he has the right to his own free will in what he does.'

I can hear the alarm bells going off in my head; I'm going to need to tread carefully.

A further meeting has been arranged and a health and safety sheet has been drafted itemising the current risks posed by some of your actions and compulsions. Falling off your walking frame has been placed in red as 'high'. A letter from the safety official at the council has arrived. Their legal department is concerned: 'Does this child have to be allowed to walk in school? We deem the risk level too high.' And I am struggling to keep things in perspective and find the words to explain that of course it is important that you walk every day in school. You don't help. You scream over and over to get into the wheelchair.

I find a solution; I design a seat that can be lowered in your frame that you can sit on. I tell you to sit down when you have the urge to hop up. And, although it makes no practical sense in stopping you from hopping, it works. But it's not allowed in school. It cannot be approved for health and safety reasons. Any attachments need to be designed and authorised by the manufacturer of the walking frame company.

'Well, do they exist? Does this manufacturer make such a seat?'

'I don't know,' comes the vague voice of the physiotherapist.

'Well, could you find out?' the headmistress asks with an exasperated voice. She's on my side at last.

And they do exist. The manufacturer does not show them in their catalogue but they will fit them on request. At the meeting the following week the physiotherapist explains she will have to write a report that will need to go to committee. It will take at least four months to get approval. And then it will have to be sent off to be fitted. My heart sinks.

'How much is it? I'll try and find the money,' I say.

The headmistress interrupts.

'Just order it, will you? I'll find the money somehow, we can't wait.'

And when it comes it is perfect for you for all sorts of reasons. You are happy again walking around the school and resting in your seat when you need to.

⌒

'Hey Louis, my number one son. I've made you lasagne!'

You squeal, doubled over in excitement.

You rang up John yesterday alerting him that you were coming. You told him you want to eat lots and lots. We have come over to Bristol again for you to have your feet checked by Mr Monsam. Now we've driven across the city to Babs, John and Adam's house. Babs is one of my oldest friends and her house is always filled with laughter. It acts as a haven, a resting point for us before making the long journey home. John is a brilliant cook and delights in feeding anyone who enters – he seems to go out of his way for us.

'I've been working on this all day for you, Lou,' John says with a broad smile as he lifts out a large bubbling glass dish.

'This is an interesting one for you, Lou. Let's see if you can tell.'

Your face has lit up, you are squealing as John is mashing up the lasagne in a bowl, adding a little cold water to cool it for you. You pick up your dessertspoon and shovel it into the bowl. You lift up a large scoop of the mashed lasagne towards your mouth – but your arm has paused. You are listening to John.

'Ooo just wait and see what I've put in this today, Louis. I wonder if you can guess?'

I jerk in my seat, say rapidly, 'John! Louis's allergies, can I check?'

'Oh, it should be all right, Al, it's Quorn and lentils,' he whispers.

'Stop, Louis!'

I knock the spoon out of your hand as it's reaching your lips; it clatters onto the wooden floor and splatters lasagne everywhere.

'I'm so sorry, John. Louis is allergic to lentils.'

'What! To lentils?'

'Yes, to lentils.'

'Oh! I thought it was nuts, peas, fish, sesame, chocolate. I didn't realise it was lentils too.'

John's got the list right. His voice is higher, he's trying

bravely to mask his disappointment. 'I'm sorry, Lou, you can't have it.'

'You've put in lentils?'

Your voice sounds incredulous.

'Yes, Lou, I didn't realise you were allergic. I'm sorry.'

'Why? Why did you do that?'

'I didn't know, Lou.'

'Why has it got lentils?'

'I didn't realise.'

'Why?'

And now whenever you hear John's name mentioned and even just out of the blue you ask that same question.

'Why did John give me lentils?'

'He didn't realise, Louis.'

'Why did he do that?'

'He didn't know.'

'Why did John put lentils in my lasagne?'

'I forgot to tell him, Lou.'

'Why . . .'

This becomes your new greeting when you meet anyone now, replacing your Phil Kay scream.

'John put lentils in my lasagne,' you tell everyone.

You have headed into puberty with us barely noticing. First

you begin to masturbate in your wheelchair when we're out and we tell you, 'No, no, Louis, not here. If you want to do that, the place to go is your bedroom.' And for once, miraculously, you are compliant. You take yourself off whenever you have the urge, into the privacy of your own room.

Greg has begun to shave you at the end of your bath time. After I've washed you and washed your hair, he comes into the room and takes over. You do not take long to develop fine stubble; there are glimmers of ginger. That must be from Greg's side; his sister Trina has magnificent orange hair that flows down to her waist. I take over again afterwards and admire your fresh face. I rub your hair with a towel a little more and help you transfer out of the bath, up onto a bench, across onto a towel-covered chair and then over into the wheelchair covered in towels and wheel you into the bedroom. I help you onto the bed and get you dressed and get your shoes on; once these are on you have the stability to walk again. I roll deodorant under your armpits; I've started to notice your manly odour when you arrive home after your exercises with David. Pimples have appeared on your back and a few on your face, not many. Your jaw has become strong and people have begun to comment on what a handsome young man you are. Your hair is thick and grows quickly. It has darkened to brown and when Daphne, our hairdresser, cuts it one day you appear like a young Liam Gallagher. You have the look of a musician about you, which of course you are.

You still think it's a compliment to invite new people you meet to take you to the bathroom. You ask them if they would like to wipe your bottom. I interrupt. I tell you again that this isn't something people enjoy doing; it's something only people who care for you, such as myself, should do. You giggle quietly to yourself. You know, don't you?

And you've started to make a frequent request for Sudocrem on your bottom. I recognise this pattern, it's got the potential to become a new obsession.

Today I'm holding your pile of maps in my hand to take out of your room and place down in the hallway. I'm raising my other hand to turn out your light.

'Goodnight, Louis, I'm off for my bike ride.'

I've closed your door but you call out for me.

'Mum, Mum, I need cream on my bottom.'

I go back in, turn the light on.

'Do you really, Louis? Are you sure?'

'Yes, yes.'

You say it urgently. Sometimes I'll agree and at other times I refuse. Today I say, 'No, Louis, I don't think that you do.'

I shut the bedroom door again, this is my third attempt to say goodnight. I'm about to call out, 'I'm off for my bike ride,' my hand is ready on the front door handle to open the door and slam but your high scream of distress has made me stop. I go back into your room again. Your cry stops.

'Okay, Louis, what is it? You can ask me one last thing.'

You have stuffed your pyjama top into your mouth. You pull it out through your clamped teeth. The top is sodden, a large wet circular patch rings around the neckline, small holes are punctured into the fabric. You are sitting up leaning against your two pillows and you turn and grin at me.

'Put some cream on my ass!'

⌒

Chantal, an artist friend, has been over to stay with her daughter Esme for a couple of days. Whenever Chantal visits I notice she gets you, really understands your concerns. When you mention your fears out loud she agrees and she's not just pretending.

'I feel like that too, Louis.'

'Yes, me too.'

'Yep, that one also.'

And you like the same food. You both love rice pudding and ice cream. 'Mmm, lasagne – that's my favourite too, Louis.'

When the time comes for Chantal and Esme to go home we take them down to the train station. You like any chance to watch trains go by. We go in our car and make promises to see each other again when we can. When we wave goodbye your hand makes hesitant jerks and as the train moves away down the track and I balance your body, turn you around to leave the station platform, my phone pings.

'I want to paint that image of you and Louis on the platform.'

A photocopy of the painting is stuck on our kitchen wall. We are standing together side by side. I am holding your hand

and have a distant look in my eye. Your tie hangs crooked and bent, the green lines of your shirt bend in the paint lines, your head is tilted and your mouth is closed but you're smiling as your eyes look directly out from the canvas.

⁓

'Why? Why did Dad scream at me?'

Greg is step-walking you into the house, looking very stressed. You are wailing your high-pitched wail, tears streaming down your face.

'Shit. That was a nightmare.'

'Why, what's happened? Don't worry, Louis, it's okay now.'

I'm trying to calm you. Your lip is down and you howl and howl.

'Why don't you go and play your piano? That will make you feel better.'

You don't move. You don't register I've said anything to you. You're sitting on the sofa stuffing your tie into your mouth then clutching your brown leather map bag tightly, making muffled screaming sounds. Your body rocks forwards and backwards as you listen.

'As we were driving into town, you know that sharp bend past those houses in Broadway? Louis pulled the door handle and the child lock wasn't on! It flew wide-open right on the bend and Louis's map case flew out. If a car had been coming the other way . . . !'

You squeeze your map case tight, making yelping sounds.

'Louis was screaming. I could see him in the mirror undoing his seatbelt; he was going to get out of the car. I was screaming at him not to. I had to slam on my brakes.'

'Oh my god, Louis, that's so dangerous. You could have been killed.'

'I ran back down the road as quick as I could to get the case, but when I turned I saw Louis had got out of the car, holding onto the doorframe in the middle of the road. A car could have come round that bend at any moment. I was screaming, "Get back in, get back in," but you didn't, did you, Louis?'

⁓

Your favourite poem right now is by John Cooper Clarke, I don't need to say which one, you know which I'm meaning. You listen to the lyrics being spoken and try to mimic them, mimic Clarke's northern nasal twang repetitively swearing. You like to finish with the words 'thank you and good night' just like on the recording.

Your interest in swearing has been creeping up for years; remember the time that your school rang us when you were eleven or twelve?

'Louis is behaving strangely today. He went with his walker into a cupboard and wouldn't come out. He used the f word too. We don't use that word in school. Have you any idea where he's got that from?'

Of course I have!

And year by year I've noticed you slipping the f word into a conversation. Not often, just every once in a while, so that you take us all by surprise and make us smile. Listen to what you said to your grandmother Mary; that one shocked even Greg. The fire was burning in the living room and you were sitting in your favourite spot on the sofa holding your maps, knowing that it was nearly time for your bedtime. Spike and Mary had been helping us that evening and were heading back to their holiday house. They'd put on their coats and Spike had already gone outside and got into the car. Mary was lingering saying kind words to you.

'It's been a lovely evening with you, Louis.'

You didn't reply – you just chewed another hole into another tie, but we all knew you were listening.

'Well, I'll be off now then, Louis. See you again soon – we're off home tomorrow.'

You are still silent.

'Have a lovely evening then, good night.'

'Of course I fucking will,' you said to our shock.

And today I've decided to go to my favourite shop with my friend Maxine. This is my occasional treat. We drive from the middle of nowhere for an hour to another middle of nowhere. Here in the most unlikely of places is the infamous Toast sale shop. Of course this means nothing to most people, but when you've lived in the middle of nowhere for as long as we have it is an enormous treat.

As I'm driving along I'm remembering our last visit to the shop. We'd got to the town and parked on the double yellow lines outside the shop. I'd helped you out of your seat and balanced you out of the car, pushed the door closed with my shoulder. We'd managed to get up the pavement and you'd held onto the handrail up the four steps into the entrance space and then I'd balanced your weight, managed to open the heavy shop door and walked you in by the arm. Phew! The armchair was free. You had looked around. There was only one other woman browsing in the shop; that was a good sign. Kirsty was standing behind the till.

'Hello, Louis, nice to see you.'

'Ah hello, Kirsty,' you shouted, thrilled. You precariously balanced over to the counter, reached out towards her breasts and then down towards her crotch with your hand, but at least you didn't quite touch.

'Louis, touch your bracelet,' I called out to you.

Kirsty mouthed over your head to me not to worry.

I got you into the armchair and I felt myself relax again. I heard the ping of the door behind as a couple came into the shop. Immediately you were holding out your hand for the man to shake and then not letting go.

'Come on, Louis, let go.'

You released his hand and stretched towards the man's crotch, looking me in the eye. If I'd said 'no' you'd do it more. I ignored you.

'Will you move away, please?' you say.

The man was leaning forwards towards you. You stretched

your hand closer towards his crotch. 'Move away.' And the man does as he's told.

'I'm sorry, he's worried about accidentally touching you.'

'Oh, okay, don't worry.'

The man turned away, looking unsurprisingly uncomfortable, studied the bargain rail then quickly left. Then you were quiet for a while. Kirsty knew just how to distract you. She came over, not too close, and asked to see your maps, took a look, then marked on one where she lived, while I nipped into the changing room, found myself a bargain dress.

You insisted on paying, you always do. You started to get worried, started to raise your voice in case I paid without you. I hauled you out of your seat and walked you up to the counter. I put my card into the machine and punched in my numbers. You shouted them out loud as I did. You know it will make people laugh.

'Shhh, Louis, don't do that. Your mum needs that to be secret.'

You looked very pleased and said the numbers aloud again. Then you pressed the green button. Kirsty pulled out the card and tore off the receipt and handed them both to you.

'There you go, Louis. Thank you very much. See you again next time, I hope.'

'Fuck you.'

'Louis!' I shouted.

I was cross with you then. This was new and disastrous

too. You'd turned away and were walking towards the door making happy whooping sounds. I shook my head and apologised as Kirsty suppressed a giggle.

'It's okay,' she said.

'No it isn't,' I'd said very loudly, 'Louis, that was very rude. If you do that again you will never be able to come in here.'

'Don't worry,' Kirsty called after us.

'I'm so sorry,' I called back as I balanced you out of the shop and down the steps towards the car as you sang the Lily Allen song out a little louder.

'Fuck you, fuck you very mu-uu-urch, I don't like what you do, I don't like your whole crew, so please don't stay in touch da da da da.'

And I've just remembered this as we are driving there today. I decide not to mention it to Maxine in case you hear and it triggers you. I hope that you have forgotten. I don't know why because you don't forget anything.

In the shop this time there's no Kirsty – it's her day off. There are two older elegant ladies who have not met you before. They've been helpful and kind and you've been good so far. And now we are paying again. Maxine is buying something from the bargain basket, a pair of corduroy trousers. She allows you to help her press the green button then one of the ladies passes you Maxine's receipt and bank card.

I hold my breath. You're not giving anything away. Will you? Won't you?

'There you go, Louis, have a nice trip home.'

You say nothing in return. You turn away and start to wobble towards the door.

'It's been a pleasure to meet you,' you call out.

The women have gasped in astonishment, 'Ah, isn't he wonderful.'

You got me again, Louis.

As I help you down the steps you giggle, 'Have I been a good boy today? Can I come here again?'

⌒

You seem rather quiet when you come in from your swimming lesson, strangely so. You go straight into your room and do not ask for a snack straight away.

'Did you have a good swim, Lou?'

You don't answer.

'Sue was cross with him this week. He touched her breasts in the water, put his hands on her wet t-shirt, so she lifted him onto the side of the pool and left him. Didn't say anything, just walked away for five minutes,' Greg says.

'Oh dear. What did she say?'

'Well, you know what she's like. She's firm. I think that it worked, kind of. I suppose it might help us. It's easier to discipline in a contained situation like that.'

'What did Lou do?'

'He just sat there on the edge, until she came back. But then he did it again. Most of his lesson was wasted. I said to Sue afterwards that really Louis just does what all of us men want to do.'

'Did you?' I laugh.

'Yes! But the way that she looked at me made me think *shit, what have I just said?*'

And I suddenly think of Barbara, our wise older neighbour and friend up in Glasgow who said to me once a long time ago, 'Louis shows us everything, all the feelings, his joy and his pain. He doesn't hide it away like we do.'

And it's true. Your tears and your laughter erupt in an instant and clearly your urges do too.

And when I think about all your current compulsions I realise your urge to touch others has always been a bit of a problem to us. Take Jack, for example: you've been touching Jack's head or shoulder for years and years. It used to be Tasha but when Jack was born you moved on to him. It's sibling rivalry in play but it is also a compulsion. Through the years Jack has had to learn to cope with it. You used to make him scream when he was young as you pulled his hair and this made you laugh. The remarkable thing is Jack's never thumped you. Even when Jack was tiny he knew you didn't understand how to behave properly, that you were vulnerable and weaker even though you hurt him. We have tried all of the obvious disciplines – taking away treats, scolding – but it's stuck as one of your long-standing compulsions. Now Jack is older he has learnt to ignore you; he realises any mention of it makes you worse.

Today, as on most days, you wheel over to Jack sitting on the sofa and place a hand on his shoulder and keep it there. Jack's had enough this time.

'Don't, Louis.'

You don't move.

'Get off me, Louis.'

You keep your hand there.

'Just get lost, will you?'

Jack moves away.

And even though you annoy him Jack is always kind to you. He lets you borrow his laptop when yours is broken. He tries to negotiate with you to make you understand not to touch him. You always agree with him.

'I promise I won't do it again,' you say.

And Jack mutters, 'But you always do.'

'I won't, I won't,' you cry as I take your maps off you again to try to teach you that you have to stop.

And you howl and howl.

But you also surprise me at times, especially when you seem to be able to turn these annoying compulsions of yours into a joke. Take yesterday, when we said goodbye to our old friends Simon and Rowan.

'Bye, Louis,' Simon said in his booming voice and stooped down to give you a hug. You put your arms around him and dug your fingers hard into his shoulders, tugged him forwards and hung onto him tight. Then it was Rowan's turn.

'Bye, Louis, see you again soon, I hope,' Rowan said in her bright high voice. She stepped forwards to hug you and you held out your arms as I balanced your body holding your hips. You put your arms around her shoulders and pulled her forwards, almost toppling her onto you.

'Piss off,' you whispered.

Rowan laughed but I heard you.

'Louis! That's not very nice. Where on earth did that come from?' I said.

'Jack,' you replied with a very pleased smile.

⁓

I've been hiding the phones from you for the last couple of years – you've asked me to help you not phone people over and over. I forget where I've put them until they ring out. Then panic ensues as we try to find them before they ring off or switch to the answering machine. But now you come home from school and play at seeking them out. You'll be screaming for me to find the landline or mobile at all costs. You know all the places I hide them, high so you can't reach, then you balance up on your legs, wobble and crash to the floor as you try to reach to the top of a shelf or the fridge, the projector, the cupboard, the wardrobe.

You want to ring Liz. I know that eventually she'll be unable to bear it. So with Liz's agreement we put into your diary the times you can call her and this instantly helps you. No longer are you searching the house over and over.

You know exactly when you can call and you stick to it like a well-designed plan.

I'm learning what's working.

Liz is a good friend. It's isolating living remotely and I'm lucky that Liz lives near here too. We've formed a close friendship and it includes you as well. She has the amazing capacity of being able to give time to you and will even have you over for sleepovers now and then. No one else but family contemplates that and you are thrilled. You've seen Tasha and Jack go for sleepovers with their friends but you've had nowhere to go. Now, every so often, Liz invites you over to stay for the night. After I've unloaded your bedding, your suitcase, your commode, your walker and wheelchair, your mashed-up food and your plastic bowl, you say to me, 'You can go now.' You've got a little independence that you enjoy. You sit in Liz's brown leather armchair in her sun room holding your maps tight and giggle as you watch her polish her kitchen floor, then you play her piano and listen as she makes her telephone calls.

'I've just had another classic from Louis,' Liz laughs down the phone. 'The window cleaner was just round. I asked him in for a cup of tea. "Would you please go now?" Louis asked him.'

'He wants you all to himself,' I laugh back.

Later, Liz calls again to tell me what time to collect you.

'You'll never believe what Louis just said to me then.'

301

'What did he say?'

'Well, I was flitting from one thought to another, speaking out loud so I could share my ideas with Louis and he said, "Liz, you are going off on a tangent!" Where on earth did he get that one from?'

And I know instantly where, and you do too, don't you?

'That's Julia, isn't it, Lou?'

Julia has been helping you for a number of years now. She is often away travelling, building her therapy business, but when she is home, back in Pembrokeshire, she offers you speech therapy with her for free. In most school holidays she invites you over to her house for a session and as the holiday season nears you excitedly ask to call her to book her into the diary. And it's not like other speech and language therapy you have experienced before. In the past the occasional hospital or school therapist has suggested you should be able to chew – 'there's nothing wrong with his jaw' – and they have tried to encourage you and me to follow their instructions and try more. Hessian sacks have been popped into your mouth with grapes inside and you've been asked to bite down, so the juice flows through, and the sack is pulled out, removed quickly before you swallow. The theory is you can learn. We've tried this on and off for years but you never do. I've now learnt there is something wrong with your bulbar muscles, the mouth and throat muscles responsible for speech and swallowing. It's through no want of trying that you don't chew or stick out your tongue, lick your lips, or blow your nose: this is all interrelated with your specific cerebral palsy condition.

But Julia does things differently, tackles the things that can help. She tries to help your speech become clearer while improving your concentration and behaviour. These are all linked: your anxiety at not being understood causes you to get in a stew before you even try to speak sometimes. Julia helps you to breathe deeply. She asks you to fill your lungs and breathe out slowly making a note, turning therapy into a song. You are enthralled as she sings out her note with a clear choir voice and you copy, singing out your note as she gently counts. It's remarkable how long you can go now. It used to be nine seconds but now it is twenty. And she's taught you some words that are fun to pronounce like 'billabong' and 'kookaroo' and then shown you on maps where Australia is, where these words come from, puts the whole thing into context for you. And she's noticed your difficulty with concentration, the way that you break off, call out in a panic. She softly calls your focus back to your game of Scrabble.

'Louis, look back at the letters – you're going off on a tangent.'

See, there it is.

And the last time I came to collect you from your special hour together I'd noticed a light in Julia's almond-shaped eyes as she opened the door.

'It was interesting and wonderful today with Louis. He demonstrated he knows what's important.'

303

I'd looked over her shoulder towards you sitting at the table squeezing your maps and biting your tie. You didn't look up or across at us.

'We've been talking about Louis's wider family. I asked him, "Who is Mary?"'

'"She's my grandmother," he answered, "she loves me very much."'

SEVENTEEN

I arrived home on Friday at midnight, crept in and up the stairs; I heard your brief cries in your fragile sleep as I passed your bedroom door. The next morning after sorting the chores, the piles of washing, I had stood in fields nearby and pushed my body into hedgerows to pull blackberries off branches. You came and watched from your seat in the car that I'd parked up close to the hedges. I'd felt thorns prick my fingers and sea air brush my face. We'd gone home with a bowl full of blackberries that I asked you to hold on your lap, as we bumped over potholes on the track. I'd rubbed flour and margarine through my fingers at the kitchen table as you'd watched from your wheelchair, whooping and biting your tie as I sprinkled the crumble-mix over the apples and berries, put two large dishes into the oven and waited until they bubbled. Every moment of our time together had felt magnified, lit up sharp and bright, our everyday actions felt alive.

'No party this year, Louis,' I explained. 'I'm sorry, it's just too complicated, Lou.' But you didn't seem to mind at all.

Julia, Maxine, Judy and Liz came over to see you later that day, and Spike and Mary, Greg, Tasha and Jack were already here too. I carried the Pyrex bowls filled with crumble and placed them onto the round wooden table outside as everyone scoured the kitchen and bedrooms, found chairs to bring out and sit on.

Greg managed you out of the front door in your walking frame and I helped to step-walk you over to sit on a sturdy chair. Your plastic bowl was filled with hot crumble and covered in copious amounts of custard as you shouted out, 'More, I'd like more, please, more.' We sat in a circle and everyone chatted and I could feel the weak autumn rays of sunshine on my back, see it lighting up faces.

And I knew I looked drawn.

Everyone was keeping the mood happy, complimenting us on the crumble we'd made and cheerfully tucking into the food with his or her spoons. I remember noticing a pale green patch of lichen growing on the outdoor table; it was lightly curling, lifting away from the table's surface, and I was transported back to my childhood, to a memory of a tattoo transfer stuck on my arm that was lifting off my skin, peeling like a lizard shedding its skin.

You didn't seem to notice I was distant, you seemed happy I'm glad to say. I'd brought you a number of Landranger maps from Edinburgh including number 169. This was one that you really wanted, and you clutched it tightly along with the other maps in your hands. You rolled the maps up and then they flapped free, and you rolled them up again. Your fingers pushed and kneaded into the covers and eventually exposed the underneath cardboard. Later that evening I stuck them all up with gaffer tape as you gave me instructions from your bed.

Once you are asleep and I'm sitting down in the living room Greg tells me you had asked him for a car for your seventeenth birthday.

'Oh no,' I answer sadly, 'what did you say?'

'I said I'm afraid that's not possible, Louis. "Why not?" Louis answered me back. Because of all of your disabilities, I'm afraid. It would be too dangerous. And do you know what he said?'

'No,' I say quietly.

'We could just try.'

Your wonderful mantra.

But you don't mention having a car to me this weekend.

As I am away from you all, new rituals form.

I must give the homeless man in the park some money, not take the bus, and later I walk the streets for hours to escape the feelings churned-up. Is that someone tailing me as I walk down the street? I pause by a window to let them pass. I cannot shake the sensation of being watched. My bag feels heavy, digs into my shoulder and my feet start to hurt and blister, but it feels better to keep moving and mull over what I've heard in this way while I'm missing you all back at home.

Because I've never been away from you for so long before. At home it'll be noisy and hectic, you'll be whooping and banging, being dressed and being fed. Here in Edinburgh it is silent, the silence is piercing; the silence is piercing my head.

I sit in a quiet café that I've found. It's become my favourite place to go at lunchtime; they make fresh simple food.

And the waitress who's served me over the weeks comes over as I stare into my soup. She's down on her knees, her head by my bowl; her bright face is looking up.

'Hi, I'm Hayley and I think that it's time that we introduced ourselves.'

My face breaks into lines of surprise. It's someone from the outside world.

'Are you a Kiwi?'

'Yes, you've got it. But what about you, what's your story?'

⌒

When are you coming home?

Tasha has sent me a text. Greg had spoken to me last night. He told me he'd seen her laptop open with a Facebook announcement, 'I miss my mum,' on the screen. Now this morning I've got this text, so there must be something up. She doesn't usually express herself like that. I phone her on her way to school.

'Are you okay, Tashi? I'm afraid I won't be back until late Friday night.'

'Oh no,' I hear her exclaim.

310

'Why, what's wrong?'

'Dad and Louis are going to have to take me then.'

'Take you where, sweetheart?'

'To Sam's house.'

'Who's Sam?'

'He's a friend.'

'Oh, is he a boyfriend?'

This will be a first.

'We don't say that, Mum; you're so old-fashioned. He's asked me over to his house for the evening.'

'Where does he live?'

'On the other side of town in a village, I can't get there without a lift. I don't want Dad and Louis to take me, but I can't get there otherwise.'

'Look, Tasha, don't worry, I'll find someone to look after Lou and then Dad can take you on his own. When is it and at what time to and from?'

Tasha's silent down the phone.

'I don't want Dad to take me either, I want you to. He'll talk to Sam's parents, knowing him.'

And that's exactly what Greg did. It turned out that Sam's mum had given Sam a message for whoever dropped Tasha off to come in for a cup of tea.

'It's like *Meet the Parents* on the first date,' Greg said. It's one of Greg's favourite films; he loves to mimic the Robert De Niro expression, 'You're in the circle of trust.'

Poor Tasha. It wasn't the best way to get to know someone, have your dad turn up with you.

When I spoke to Greg later that evening after he'd brought Tasha home and you were asleep in bed he sounded happy.

'Sam's a cool kid, we got on great.'

'Greg! That was supposed to be Tasha's date.'

I can picture the scene. It was just what Tasha had known was going to happen.

⌒

I've missed your school Christmas fête because of being up here in Edinburgh. Greg takes you instead.

'That was hard work,' he tells me down the phone. 'Louis was obsessing about seeing Father Christmas. He made a beeline for the grotto in his walking frame. I was holding tight onto the back bar pulling him back from knocking over other children in the queue. He wouldn't wait.'

I can picture it all; I've been there before. Each year you come up with something obscure that you want for Christmas and get overexcited. Last year you wanted a Sound Beam, repeatedly asking for one. I knew what one was as there was one in your school. It consists of a number of poles on stands with movement sensors that are positioned around you and if you move parts of your body invisible sound beams sense these movements and translate them into sounds. You rarely get to use it in school as it requires the music teacher who is only in once a week and there are other children who benefit from this equipment much more than you do, but you love it when you do get a go.

I researched the cost of a Sound Beam and it was thousands of pounds so I told you over and over again it wasn't possible to have this for Christmas, but you didn't seem to understand. One day you called me into your bedroom and showed me your computer screen; you'd sent a letter to Santa via a Santa website all on your own and had got a reply.

Ho Ho Ho, Louis, it's nice to hear from you and you say you've been a good boy, well done Louis, well done. My my my Louis you are getting to be a big boy now, sixteen years old I see. What is this that you say that you want, A Sound Beam? Ho Ho Ho I will try. But oh dear me, I see you say you'll be sad if you don't get one. Now my ears always prick up when I hear words like that. You must talk to an adult about your feelings . . . Ho Ho Ho and a very Merry Christmas to you, Louis. I'll try my best to fit what you want in my sleigh.

You'd been watching my face as I read. This was something new for you, to look for an emotional response in me. As I finished reading I looked over to you and you cried out.

'He will try.'

'But Louis, it's too expensive.'

But you just giggled with joy.

I did Internet searches but there was nothing second-hand and then I had a brain wave and rang the Sound Beam Company to see if they had any old equipment for sale. They said no, it was rare for their equipment to come up second-hand. I was about to ring off when the woman interrupted my goodbye.

'Wait a minute. I don't like the idea of your son being disappointed on Christmas Day. I'll need to check with my boss, but as we close over Christmas and New Year I'll ask if we could lend you one of our demo sets over the Christmas holidays.'

I was amazed at her offer.

Last year you opened a box on Christmas Day and squealed in delight. There was a Sound Beam. You didn't mind at all that it had to be returned shortly after.

'What did Louis ask for this time?' I ask Greg.

'He asked for a hot tub.'

'What! A hot tub!' I laugh. 'Where has that come from?'

'He said Mrs Philips has one in her garden.'

Mrs Philips is one of the learning support assistants in your classroom. She is lovely. She has a radiant face, a warm personality and very large bosoms. She is always extremely complimentary about you.

Greg continues, 'Then when we got home the other kids heard what Louis had asked for and they agreed that they want one too.'

'So what do you think?'

'There's no way we're getting a hot tub. We can't afford a decent one and a cheap one will break, that's for sure.'

⌣

When I do get home for Christmas this year I'm afraid you don't get the hot tub you asked for. I have managed to collect an enormous number of Landranger OS maps from the Oxfam shop in Edinburgh. You are perfectly happy when you discover these are your main present on Christmas Day. We put up a second shelf in your bedroom and place all your maps in numbered order, and then we make a list of all the ones you still have to collect; you're doing rather well, we see, when we look at the list.

You don't mention the hot tub you asked for at all, thank goodness.

⌣

It's New Year's Day morning and I can hear you're awake in your bedroom as I come downstairs to dress you and give you your breakfast. I open your door.

'Louis, do you want to go down to Little Haven and watch the New Year's Day swim? Dad might do it.'

'Yes,' you say back.

'You'll need to be quick,' Greg calls down the stairs, 'it's at nine thirty this year.'

'You go ahead with Tasha and Jack, I'll catch you up with Louis,' I call back.

The old car door slams and Greg speeds off down the drive; he doesn't want to miss the beginning and neither do I, but it takes time, it always takes time to do all the preparations to get you ready.

I lift the wheelchair into the car boot, make sure your coat is zipped up tight, then we follow Greg's route down to the village. As we come down the steep hill, turn the corner towards the seafront there's a crowd at the wall and a number of people I recognise, some in their swimming costumes, standing ready to go into the sea on the slip. I see Andy Grey ready with his loudspeaker and horn as we drive by and up to the car park. I hoick the wheelchair out of the boot and wheel it around to the passenger door, take the bunch of maps from your hands and tuck them under my arm trying not to drop them as I undo your car buckle. You make no attempt to move.

'Come on, Louis, we'll miss it,' I encourage you. You sit still, chewing the top of your coat and just as I'm losing hope you respond, lean forwards and move your legs round. I take your weight as you lean onto my shoulders and slide your legs down out of the car to the ground, and I try to pull the chair closer without falling as you manage to sit down. I buckle you in and pull the footplates down and turn you around and start to push you towards the seafront. You're getting heavier I notice. Will we make it in time? Not quite. I hear the horn blasting as we're heading down the short road to the sea. We reach the seafront but can't see over the crowd at the wall, so I turn and push you up to the left past the Swan Inn to look down on the beach from a higher viewpoint. I have to push hard to get you up the hill and eventually find a free space along the wall to push your chair up close to it. Then you put on your brakes and I take your maps again and help pull you up and out to lean and look over the wall down into the water. There in the sea are some swimmers dressed up in fun outfits, splashing around, but most are running out of the water back up the slipway, their bodies rose pink from the cold.

'Did you see Dad go in, where's he now?' I ask Tasha and Jack who've appeared with their friends Zak and Jamie by our side on the wall. They both stretch out their arms and point down.

'There he is,' Tasha says.

Greg's already out of the sea and is standing with a towel around his waist and a puffy coat over his torso; he is mingling in the crowd on the slipway chatting to any and everyone, as he does. So I wheel you back down the hill and into the friendly crowd to chat with friends and neighbours, and Jamie's mum Elaine kindly crouches down to look at your maps with you.

⌒

The Christmas and New Year holidays are over and I have to force myself to leave you all again to return to Edinburgh.

⌒

I'm home at last in the week as well as weekends. Natasha has her GCSE exams coming up which I feel dreadful about, she's needing help and support with her work, and Greg needs me to take over fast – he's got work to get on with. He's been designing a park for the Commonwealth Games in Glasgow. This creative commission is a big piece of luck to have come our way on the back of our reputation from years ago in Scotland. Now down in Wales any design work has mostly dried up. The job came in last summer and it could not have come at a better time for keeping our heads above water. So the moment that I get home Greg is off to Glasgow to check the construction work is being done correctly.

Unsurprisingly the house is a tip; there are piles of paperwork and washing to sort out, all your care needs to see to, a review to attend at your school, a hospital appointment with your paediatrician, the tax returns to finish, and the list goes on and on.

⌒

It is late February and my younger sister Jenny is coming down to visit us. It will be some wonderful light relief.

Jenny had a baby in November, a baby girl named Lyra, and she's going to come from Manchester and visit us all with the new baby. I can't wait to see them both. Tasha's excited too but Jack's not impressed. He finds babies annoying, he tells me.

And what will you make of the baby? You are used to having Jenny all to yourself; it will be a bit of a shock now she's become a mother.

You come down to the train station to pick them both up.

Jenny wisely sits in the back of the car between you and the baby. She has to protect Lyra from your swipes on the journey back to our house. When we get home Jenny carries the baby into the house and I balance you up onto your feet out of the car, tuck your maps under my armpit and step-walk you into the house too.

Jenny's settled herself down on the sofa and has Lyra in her arms.

'Hey Louis, what do you think of the baby?' Jenny asks you.

Right on cue you give her your answer, with an enormous wide smile on your face. You've not forgotten Colin's expression.

'The baby's a pain in the ass.'

You've started to hit your head hard and, like all your compulsions, it has been building for a number of years, but whereas before we could live with it (it was only a light tap with your head on a table) now it's a full whack. When you wheel yourself up to the table I quickly put my hand down over the wooden edge. You bring your head down hard on my palm then you lean your head from side to side trying to hit the sharp edge while I cushion each thump. Eventually your urge subsides and you stop, but I can't protect you all of the time. When you go to the toilet I hear to my horror a ceramic clunking sound as you head-butt the sink, and you've begun to raise your fists up to your head to hit your forehead with your knuckles. When anyone sees you they tell you to stop and you scream and respond by hitting yourself over and over. So we've all gone silent and instead we try to distract you.

I've found foam matting and have cut it into squares and stuck the pieces around the house as safety precautions and I've bought lots of headbands and inner boxing gloves to wear on your hands. These are padded at the knuckles to protect your head from your fists. It's not ideal; I know this new look will stick and I miss the old you, but it's far too risky not to protect you at the moment.

You love all these solutions. You take a foam mat with you everywhere and you wear your headband and gloves all day long and only agree to take them off at night-time. As I head for your bedroom door to turn off your light I hear the sound of your fists as you whack yourself a few times as you lie there.

In the morning you sit at the kitchen table having breakfast. I see you lift up your headband, whack your head on the edge of table then quickly pull it back down.

'There's no point in wearing the headband if you do that,' Greg tells you firmly and you hold onto the headband tight.

'I'll take it off you.'

'No, no, no,' you call out.

And today I've found someone who may be able to help with your compulsions. It's Jack Woods who runs the disabled basketball class that you go to. Jack's noticed your increased hitting.

'What's up with Louis?'

'It's a compulsion. It's best to ignore it or he does it more.'

'Right, but do you know why he's doing it? It looks painful.'

'I think he's frustrated.'

'Maybe I could help, I do music therapy.'

'You do?' I'm incredulous. 'Louis learnt to speak through music.'

'Oh, right. Well, I'd love to help in the future if I get any time.'

Jack Woods calls to say he's found time for an hour of music therapy one evening a week. He comes over to our house with a drum and a stand. He talks to you in your room on your own and we hear drum beats as you compose your own song, beat it out in rhythmic time. I hear crescendos in the music and then it goes quiet. Jack's explaining how to meditate through deep breathing. Our house has become hushed; you've briefly gone silent and still.

This could work.

This is what you need in your life, others who can befriend you, understand and help you as you go into adulthood.

⁓

I'm looking forward to my lie in. There's no reason for me to have to get up early today because your school has an

INSET day. As I went to bed last night I made a mental note. I'm going to try to block out your noises from downstairs for as long as I can; if I'm lucky I'll not have to get up until nine to dress you and give you your breakfast. Hopefully you'll get preoccupied on your computer and I might get away with it. I'm tired tonight.

I've left my mobile phone on a chair that holds a light by my side of the bed, I've turned off the ringer but I've not put it on silent. At six thirty it buzzes. *Oh what?* It buzzes again. I can hear your quiet whoops from beneath the floorboards, hear the creak of the wheelchair. The text is from Sue Grainger, someone I know a little.

'R u aware that Louis has posted your and Greg's pin numbers on Facebook?'

What! I bolt upright. Greg groans, 'What is it? You've woken me up.'

I'm out of the bedroom and down the stairs and into your room. You are sitting in your wheelchair by your table looking at your computer. As I open your door I see your finger press a key and a page on your screen disappears.

'Louis, what are you doing?'

You are briefly silent, then you pull your pyjama top out of your mouth. 'Nothing,' you say.

'Yes you are. I've just had a text from Sue Grainger. You've put our pin numbers on Facebook.'

You chew your pyjama top and stay silent.

'Louis? Have you done that?'

'Yes.'

'Well, you mustn't, you know that. We need to take them off immediately.'

I don't do Facebook but lots of my family and friends do and it is great for you. It keeps you occupied; you send people messages and people send nice messages back. I don't know how to navigate around the thing.

'Louis, you need to show me what you've done.'

You've already reopened your Facebook page: I can't see anything there.

'Have you deleted it?'

'Yes.'

I go back upstairs to the bedroom, text Sue. 'Thanks for telling me. Louis says he's deleted it, has he?'

I slip into bed and close my eyes, the phone buzzes, I look at the screen: 'No, it's still there.'

I'm back down the stairs.

'Louis, it's still there, show me,' but I can't find it on your screen. You seem to have deleted it from what I can tell but it is still posted as a newsfeed to all of your friends. I call Jenny; it's gone seven now and she's driving to work.

'Jen, Louis's put our pin numbers on Facebook. How do I get them off?'

'Oh shit, has he? I'll call you when I get to work.'

Jenny takes me through the paces to delete it completely from the system.

'Yes,' Sue texts me at eight. 'It's gone now.'

I've given up on sleeping. Greg's disappeared from my side

and has gone downstairs to make himself a cup of tea, but I lie up here contentedly resting, stretching out my limbs in the bed. I know if I get up my footsteps will trigger you off, you will start to call out instructions for me to get you dressed. I want a little bit longer of this peace. Your computer will keep you occupied for a while longer I'm hoping.

I can hear certain sounds beneath me so I've guessed what is coming; this is your new favourite game when you look at your screen. You've turned the sound up, this is always a sign, and yes, I am right, you are on YouTube. I can hear the creaking and rumbling, the clanking of metal, distant voices chattering and then there's a silence, a long pause, here goes, you are shouting, screams echo out from your room, happy screams from others in fear and the sound of the wheels whooshing down across metal. Your voice is deeper, you are shouting, 'Ahhhhhhh, ahhh, ahhh, ahhhhhhhhh,' and your throat sounds hoarse, then you switch to your new favourite cry, you shout loudly at the top of your voice, 'Stop the ride, stop the ride, stop the ride.'

Thank goodness the campsite is not open right now. I do sometimes wonder what our campers think as they lie in their tents in our field. What do they make of the distant strange noises that sometimes drift out of our house?

I decide to get up.

As my feet touch the floorboards you stop shouting 'Stop the ride,' and call out, 'Mum, Mum, Mum, get me dressed,' and I hear your wheelchair turning to the bedroom door as I walk down the stairs.

This is the fifth social worker in the last eight months: they keep leaving. They all say the same thing but only after I've had to describe our situation to them in great detail. Then they agree that I'm using the direct payments awarded wisely. The payments are not enough to go round, there's a shortfall and I make up the difference with the help of a trust fund set up by your great-aunt Alison with money from family and friends who care about you.

The direct payments go on exercise and activities like physio and swimming. After explaining to each social worker they always agree that what we are doing is necessary for us all. That without this exercise you'd likely be in a wheelchair permanently, which would increase your care needs, that your obsessional behaviour would get worse if you had nothing to do.

I find these meetings exhausting and I'm worried. You are about to turn eighteen and none of the social workers I've seen so far can tell me what this will mean. Will they take this current funding away? And what about the overnight respite we get one day a week, will it continue?

I've been phoning and phoning the social work department to ask what will happen, and each time I'm told that our last social worker has left. Now today I have a meeting with our latest assigned social worker, called Felix.

Felix walks into our kitchen and my hopeful heart sinks. He's looking around assessing the way that we live and the way that he does feels intrusive. The downstairs of our house consists mostly of one long room and from Felix's chair in the kitchen he can see the wood burner at the far end of the living room, the sofas and television, the filled bookshelves and into Greg's music space, a table and instruments scattered, and then into the kitchen where Greg's wall of favourite pictures are pinned.

'That's a large bag of rice,' Felix says.

'I'm sorry?'

'That's a large bag of rice you've got.'

Oh no, is he going to be useless?

Felix has turned to look out of the kitchen window. 'Who lives in the caravan?' he asks.

'We haven't got a spare room, it acts as somewhere for visitors.'

'You have apples on that tree.'

'Yes, we do.' I take a deep breath, this man is stalling, he seems as unsure of being here as I am.

'Can we talk about Louis and his needs?' I say directly. 'I'm worried, really worried about him turning eighteen in two weeks. What's going to happen to the respite and the direct payments then? Will they continue or do they suddenly stop?'

'Ah yes. Well, the respite will finish. There's nothing for adults.'

I take an intake of breath. 'Nothing at all?'

'No. There used to be but it's been cut, there's not any more.'

Felix's narrow face is pale. He raises his fair eyebrows and taps his pen on his diary.

'So how do adult services work?' I ask him.

He shrugs his shoulders.

'Well, I don't know the answer to that. You will be seen again by an adult services social worker. I've got to write a report on you now, sign you over. You should have been seen by the transition social worker but she's been off sick for the last six months. We're a bit behind.'

'So where does that leave us now?'

'Is that a saxophone?'

'Sorry?'

'Is that a saxophone you've got there?'

Oh bloody hell.

~

You are excited about your upcoming birthday. You tell us you will no longer need Judy, that instead you will be coming out with us, you will be coming down to the pub you say gleefully, you are going to be an adult so you will not need looking after at all any more. I don't know where all this knowledge has come from about being eighteen but it takes me by surprise that you comprehend its significance so well. I'm having trouble knowing how to answer you without dampening your enthusiasm and joy.

'Yes of course, Louis, you can come out with us sometimes, but not always. Sometimes me and Dad need a bit of time on our own. It's not really to do with age.'

'But I'll be eighteen,' you respond.

'Of course I'll take you out to the pub one night,' Greg answers with a chuckle. And that's all you want to hear right now.

EIGHTEEN

Today it's your eighteenth birthday.

A year has passed, a year that has felt like a lifetime condensed into one. A year that has stretched us further than I realised we could ever be stretched.

The intervening year is held as balls of lead in my head and my heart. I'm peppered with bullets and I don't know how to begin to explain what's occurred.

Today it's your eighteenth birthday and I'm focusing wholly on that. I must keep the memories away, keep them out of our life.

As you turn eighteen, as we were told, our respite has been cut to nothing, gone. Yesterday you were a child and today you are an adult and everything will change with social services again but nothing has changed with you. You still need all of your care, but nobody seems to be able to tell us anything.

We are not going to worry. We are having a party and your parties are known as the best. You have been calling people up over the last few weeks, inviting them to come to our house on Sunday afternoon to celebrate. Anyone you have met over the years is invited. You don't remember that you've not seen some of them for a very long time; you just remember that they have come to one of your parties before.

'How many are coming?' Greg asks.

'I'm really not sure.'

Squidge is coming and is going to tune your sitar and Alex is coming along with his tambura to play. Yes, you've met someone around here who can play one of those. All sorts of friends and family will arrive who have loved, helped and cared for you over the years. Our lives would be so much bleaker without these friendships and instead it feels rich today. It's filled with the generosity of others who are prepared to come and spend time with you.

Dan the Man's come down from the Midlands to be at your birthday party. Dan used to live near here a few years ago. He was the manager at the local theatre and cinema house that we visit and would let you go up and down, up and down, repeatedly, again and again in the lift.

And here comes our good friend Lorraine through the front door carrying a very large box in her arms. She's made great efforts to be here today, has come all the way over from Dorset.

'Will you give me a bath?' you call out in your deepened voice as soon as you see her. Lorraine used to help bath you when you were small.

'Ooo, Louis, you're a big boy now!' Lorraine answers in her *Carry On* voice. And you giggle with joy at your naughty suggestion. When you open the lid of her box you beam wide with delight: it's eighteen tins of your favourite Ambrosia rice pudding. And now Judy and Dick have arrived. Judy clutches something wrapped up in her hand.

'I thought this might help Louis at the moment.'

Judy's always so kind. When she takes you to swimming

or to boccia she'll come back to our house with ideas. This time it's a knitted headband with a fleecy lining inside.

'For the winter,' she says.

You like it! If you hadn't you'd have dropped it on the floor, forgotten it instantly. But you don't; instead you whip off your tennis headband and pull the knitted one over your head right down to your eyes.

And for the first time at a party you have three other young people here with special needs. You take no notice of them at all until Gerallt, who is younger and has Down's syndrome, decides to sit behind you on your favourite armchair and try to push you off. Then you shout at him to 'go away', as you clutch your maps and chew your tie. Adults mill around you drinking wine, laughing, and the sound of a sitar being played filters from out of your bedroom.

And then Saskia arrives.

She strides into the people-filled living room, tall and slender in her ballerina skirt, her blond hair tied up high. She marches up to me as I pour drinks in the kitchen.

'You are Louis's mum,' she says with an imperious voice.

'Yes, I am. Hi, Saskia.'

'Where's the cake? It's mine.'

'Yes, Saskia, that's fine.'

She strides away and Leonie, her mother, comes and whispers.

'Let me know when you are going to light the candles. Saskia will scream. I'll have to take her out of here.'

I've been inviting Leonie and Saskia to our house for the last couple of years. I felt she could be a potential friend, that we would understand each other's predicament too, but it's not been possible until today.

'I was amazed when I saw you come in.'

'Well, I'm rather amazed too. Saskia's been stamping her feet all week in a rage saying, "It's my birthday, not Louis's." But then Saskia got up this morning and made me write "It's Saskia's Birthday" on the big whiteboard in our kitchen. As soon as I did she announced, "We're going to Louis's house now."'

I hardly ever speak with other parents with disabled children about what we are trying to cope with day by day. We usually can't stand still talking if the children are with us, but Saskia seems to be settling in; Greg's taken her under his wing.

'Our respite's ended today.'

I regret saying this as I see Leonie's shoulders turn in.

'I can't even contemplate that,' she says, looking at me with her beautiful but haunted eyes. 'I've got another six months, then I don't know what I'll do.'

'I'm sorry I mentioned it. Let's not think about it today. Can I get you a drink?'

So we celebrated your eighteenth birthday surrounded by noise and laughter. Saskia pretended your birthday was hers, she told everyone so and you didn't even notice, you really didn't care. She commanded when to light the candles, and held the cake while they burned. Leonie kept her distance and widened her eyes with amazement as our gazes caught. As we all sang, Saskia crouched over as if doubled up in pain but she managed to stay stationary, not run away when everyone cheered.

'We might be able to come here again!' Leonie whispered as they left shortly after.

I can hear you speaking loudly somewhere behind me as I stand by the open front door. You don't seem to be able to control your voice level but it's mostly understandable now. You are talking to David.

'Can we go to Dina's Head next time?'

'Where, Louis? I've not heard of there.'

'Dina's Head.'

'Where's that then, Louis?'

You pause. 'I don't know.'

'Has somebody told you about it?'

'Yes. Aiden at Holly House.'

That's the respite centre you can no longer attend.

'Ah, well, maybe. I'll have to speak with your mum. Do you know if it's far away?'

'Yes.' You draw out the 'e' and the 's'.

'It's a bit of a drive, it's up near Fishguard,' I call out over my shoulder.

'Ah, I see, Louis. I'll have to see.'

'Yes,' you say as your mouth opens wide, showing your teeth.

'I might need more time to take you there.'

'Yes,' you say louder with an enormous grin.

'I'll have to try and plan it. I'll have to see what I can manage.'

'Just try,' you say, doubling over with laughter, squealing with delight, knowing that David will.

⁓

I experience an overwhelming feeling of tenderness towards you on your birthday. I feel it flood into my veins when I see you come in through our open front door. You are being pushed in your wheelchair; you don't notice my swollen eyes. You are beaming; you've had fun being taken out in John's car. You have no understanding of the enormous significance of this day and what it means for your future. Greg is exceptionally gentle towards you too; I notice the change in his voice. Is it linked to our sense of life and death? At least you are safe with us now.

EPILOGUE

A few months after Louis's birthday he got an infection in his right foot and lost the ability to walk for four months. It took two visits to the GP and four to A&E to eventually work out what was wrong. His feet are so twisted it was difficult for the doctors to diagnose the cause. Louis worried he might never be able to walk again but with three courses of medication and special exercises from David, we have got Louis back onto his feet again.

I have addressed my memoir to Louis, although he would not be able to comprehend what I have said in any meaningful way. He may enjoy parts like the Phil Kay section, although he's stopped screaming about Phil right now; instead Louis's current favourite greeting is to gleefully cry, 'I put my mum and dad's pin numbers on Facebook.' He revels in delight at the shocked responses he gets.

This story is also Greg, Natasha and Jack's. I have tried to respect their privacy as much as I can. This is why you may wonder at times where they have gone in the story. Greg hasn't read the memoir. He says he doesn't need to: he's lived it. I hope anyone reading can see that Greg has been trying incredibly hard, for an incredibly long time.

This story is also about our family and friends who have stood by us and helped us through the years, especially Spike and Mary, my parents. Both Greg and I acknowledge they have saved us many times. There are others who should be in this story. I'm sorry if I've missed you out, your support has also been important to us.

This story is written from memory. These moments are seared on my brain. I let my mind choose which ones would erupt for me to write down. They came out in a jumbled torrent and it feels good that they are now on the page. I can let go; let the future come into our lives. Of course, I must point out that the dialogue is from memory so won't be completely accurate. But the conversations capture my impression of the moments and perception of what was said.

This memoir is about a mother's love for her son. It is also about hope – hope in others, hope in systems, and hope for the future. It is about sharing, trying, wanting and giving. It is what all of us humans need and feel.

The future is frightening. I worry about Louis and his care requirements all the time. Greg and I are tired and getting older. How much more energy do we have left?

I'm aware when I say this that we are not in any way unique or different from all the others who are struggling; we are more fortunate than many with all the help and support we've been given.

Service cuts make me worried for all of our futures. When I heard the other week that Holly House, the children's respite centre close to us, is facing cuts my heart froze. It saved us in our time of extreme need, when Louis was waking seven times in the night. What will happen for others like us? I hope this story can help others to comprehend how tragic it will be to lose places like this. We parents need voices in high places to prevent such a terrible thing.

When Louis turned nineteen I discovered that Greg had called social services and told them we could no longer cope. I was horrified and worried what would happen to Louis but it turns out that Greg did the right thing. At last we were assigned a social worker who knew her job. We were given hours of respite with an amazing new organisation called Value Independence. Since being given this help Louis's outlook has begun to seem brighter. Value Independence is a social enterprise company that wants to help adults with disabilities have as much independence and active fun as they can. It's remarkable it exists at all. Its vision is great, its monetary means small, but the staff are doing wonderful things with Louis. Louis gets to say what he wants to do and they try to make it happen. As you can imagine, Louis comes up with all sorts of suggestions: 'I want to see a steam train,' 'I want to do a bungee jump,' 'I want to post a letter to Oonagh,' 'I want to go for a shave at Bromos' (the barbers – Louis wants to avoid having a bath at home later), 'I want to visit a radio station.' There is always something that Louis has thought of to try, and, thanks to Value Independence, Louis has been having a ball.

Last autumn as Louis turned twenty some more good news came our way; amazingly after a three-year application process Louis has been given the chance of attending a residential educational college. There he can have music therapy, enjoy drama and exercise and integrate with others his age. Louis was nervous about this major life change but wanted to go. There's been little for him to do back at home with school having finished. The Welsh Government and our local council have agreed funding for two or possibly three years and he started college a few months ago. Needless to say, it was quite a preparation process and I was in emotional turmoil as I drove Louis and all of his things to the college, but it was Louis who helped me at that moment. As he scooped cake and custard into his mouth at the service station en route to the college I told him I was going to miss him and he paused as he ate, held his spoon in the air and told me with an expectant face, 'It's all part of growing up.' It's at that moment I realised that Louis has all the same wishes and desires that we all have, he needs a little independence by his age. Now he's gone he's still keeping me on my toes from afar with his mischief (there's more stories) and comes home for long periods to be with us in the holidays, and of course will be back with us when college finishes.

Finally, this story is offered as a glimpse of our lives. I've never quite known where to begin when someone asks me what I've been up to. I've never quite known how to explain what our daily life is like. I wanted to write how it is in order to give others a greater understanding of disability and caring. And to be totally honest, I wanted to write something that would make people consider being Louis's friend, or a friend to some other mentally and physically disabled person. It's worth it, it's a challenge, but it definitely makes you feel like you are alive.